WALKING MIRACLE:

LIVING WITH A CHRONIC ILLNESS

ADVANCE CARE PLANNING RESOURCES

Richard Tucker

Walking Miracle: Living with a Chronic Illness. Advance Care Planning Resources

For permission requests, send an email to the copyright owner Email: info@mbtstrategies.com Ordering Information: Quantity sales, Special discounts are available on quantity purchase by corporations, associations, and others. For details, contact the publisher info@mbtstrategies.com Orders by U.S. trade bookstores and wholesalers, please contact Marilyn Bryant-Tucker: (919) 345-2892 Printed in the United States of America Book Design and Layout by Marilyn Bryant-Tucker, Owner of MBT Marketing Solutions & Associates www.mbtstrategies.com

ISBN: 9781660176052

Dedication

I would like to dedicate this book to my wife, Marilyn. I would like to thank her for her support and encouraging me. I never could have made it without her.

Acknowledgements
From The Co - Author

To my Mother Lossie Dupree, thank you for being right by my side to weather the **storm.**

Thanks to all the medical staff, family, friends and past co-workers for all your support and prayers.

Table Of Contents

Introduction

A book of this nature is not a marital vow or anything that has to do with holy matrimony. But the reason the book could be written owes its life to the biblical saying finding a good wife. This book by Richard Tucker co-authored by Marilyn Bryant Tucker is a testimony to the word of God about finding a good wife. The book of proverbs 18:22 (NKJV) says: "He who finds a wife finds a good thing, and obtains favor from the Lord."

The Advance Care Planning Resources Book has a four-prong objective. It is carefully planned to give the reader a ray of hope and a guide when life challenges beckon.

The objectives are

- To serve as your guide to overcome life-threatening health conditions

- The need for excellent family life, especially a caring spouse

- To admonish the reader to lead a healthy lifestyle when in wholesome health

- To make God and His words your guide throughout your life activities

This book reminds us that we are a living creation of nature accountable for the things we do. How we live, what we do, and how we do it all have a way of getting back at us. We are also blessed to have people who shared their experiences of encounters with chronic illness. While its aim to give us strength in troubled times, its goal is to prepare us for a life of challenge.

Walking Miracle reports the journey of Richard Tucker in his battle with serial chronic illnesses. He fought, chiefly with diabetes, heart disease, kidney failure and loss of peripheral vision. He is a man qualified to claim to make a return journey from the land of the dead on several occasions. He survived battles with strokes, heart attacks, and cardiac arrest more than once; he is a customer of ER, life support and ICU. Richard Tucker had suffered Congestive Heart Failure (CHF) and peripheral vision crises, and to the glory of God, he lives to tell the story.

This book is not another medical literature full of professional jargon. It is a contribution from a family that went through the trouble of self-rescue from the clutches of death! There are several medical books on the health conditions being through by Richard already. Therefore, the Advance Care Planning Resources Book is not to repeat any of their recommendations. However, this book is to serve as your co-walker through the shadows of death. It will walk with you to overcome your challenges. It is to remind you that there is light at the end of the tunnel.

Incidentally, Richard Tucker is a man full of life! In him is a man of exceptional character who wants to live life on his terms. He loves his black Dodge Ram, have coffee with workmates in morning meeting and live a life of an entrepreneur. Mr. Tucker is a happy family man who loves and cherishes his wife and grateful to God for her life.

However, health challenges began to threaten his sweet lifestyle when he was diagnosed in 1997with high blood pressure! Not many, who went through the experience of Richard in his encounter with chronic illness, live to tell the story. Therefore, the Advance Care Planning Resources Book, co-authored by him and his darling wife, Marilyn Bryant Tucker, is his way to appreciate God for life.

With firsthand experience of chronic illnesses, Richard and Marilyn decided to share useful information in Walking Miracle. The book is written to be fun and easy to follow. Perhaps, as you read, you will resonate with some of the facts shared as evident in your own life.

Some of the chapters in the book that will make exciting read include:

- **FAMILY**. Books this nature celebrates the role and value of family in health care management. Sometimes, when the vital first aid from close people is missing, not many live to tell the story of recovery.

- **CONGESTIVE HEART FAILURE**. It is a medical term for heart failure, and this topic talks about causes and prevention. Richard understands better how a simple lifestyle change could have prevented the long-suffering and safe the family avoidable health expenses.

- **FIRST RESPONDERS**. When someone suffers a heart attack or involved in a medical emergency, there is a need for immediate medical attention to resuscitate and manage the patient before the arrival of qualified medical personnel. This book discusses the importance of family member acquiring such skills to save lives.

- **PALLIATIVE CARE**. Every human problem requires adequate response to manage both real and side effects of life-threatening illness. The book explains the real meaning of palliative care and its application in walking through chronic disease.

- **ADVANCE CARE PLANNING**. Richard learned a big lesson from his experience with life support and ICU cases while receiving treatment for his chronic illness condition. Readers would learn the importance of deciding while in health to make it easy to care for you in a life-threatening situation when you can least choose.

- **FAITH and GOD**. When you are in a crisis, it may look like the world is going to end soon, but for the believers in God, their hope knows no limit. God is the alpha and omega who knows the unknown, and when medical science failed, spiritual belief will save the day. The importance of this discussion is that being a God believing family, Richard and Marilyn know that there is the unseen hand sustaining them. Many have died for far less chronic illness; therefore, readers are encouraged to give faith and believe in God when facing life-threatening health condition.

- **COMPLIANCE**. Compliance is technically about safe and high-quality care for patients. It is not only the responsibility of health institutions to comply; the individual must live to ensure wholesome health free of ailments and diseases. While health organizations follow the code of ethics in ensuring patient safety, the patient needs to play its part in helping to achieve success in their care.

There are other interesting topics in the Advance Care Planning Resources Book every reader will find quite interesting to read. Mr. Tucker's experiences of his encounter with life-threatening diseases in a book are worth reading.

Congestive Heart Failure

I was diagnosed with high blood pressure in 1998 and prescribed blood pressure pills, but I did not follow the prescription. While I was working a few weeks later at milk containers for the company, I could not do at work. My routine job consisted of lifting boxes; these were empty milk carton, but I found it difficult moving them. I had to take permission to go home to rest due to fatigue.

On February 14, 1998, which was a Valentine's Day, I was diagnosed with congestive heart failure (CHF). Before being diagnosed with CHF, I had thought it was cold. For several weeks, I was taking over the counter medicine and drinking hot tea because the symptoms were similar to that of a cold.

There and then, the Doctor prescribed me Lasix.

Lasix (aka furosemide) is a loop diuretic (water pill) that prevents your body from absorbing too much salt. This allows the salt passed in your urine. It is for the treatment of fluid retention (edema) in patients suffering from liver disease, kidney disorder (Nephrotic Syndrome) or congestive heart failure.

I took Lasix from 1998-2008. At times my wife would have to meet me to pop a pill in my mouth to get rid of fluid or feel better.

Incidentally, the Office of the Doctor I was attending closed and my Doctor moved to a hospital. As a result of that, I started seeing a new Doctor between 2008 and 2016; that was for eight good years. She took me off Lasix because she said it could damage my kidneys. It was during this time frame I had a heart attack (2008), and congestive heart failure flares up (2013); I came down with cardiac arrest and stroke in (2015).

I was not knowledgeable about congestive heart failure, but I am today. I know the importance of eating a low sodium diet, no added salt, walking, not smoking, and taking my medications. I stopped drinking in my twenties, so that was not an issue.

As you can see, my condition was as a result of ignorance of the developmental processes of a heart condition. Therefore, I have resolved to share some knowledge with people to help them avoid heart condition, including CHF.

Causes and management of congestive heart failure

The chronic progressive heart health condition called Congestive Heart Failure (CHF) affects the pumping power of the heart muscles. Also, CHF is called "heart failure," and it happens when fluid accumulates around the heart leading to inefficient pumping. There are four heart chambers with two atria at the upper half and two ventricles at the lower half. Each half performs pumps (ventricles) and receives (atria) blood to and from the body organs. After progressive chronic heart health, the point at which the ventricles fail to pump sufficient blood to the body is when CHF develops.

It may sound incredible that about 5.7 million American adults have heart failure, but it's true! My experience battling CHF and real-life account from my wife left me with goose pimples about the experience. It is not the pain alone; you can imagine the costs which stood at $30.7 billion annually. Well, if the material cost isn't enough to prevent heart failure, you need to know that half of CHF sufferers die within five years of being diagnosed. Think of the immediate, medium and distant result of CHF, and you would prefer to stay off its radar for your own good.

Once you discover you are suffering congestive heart failure, the next thing is management. I have learned a great lesson from my lackadaisical attitude in handling the events that followed the news of my CHF condition. I am blessed to have my wife, who care more than anything in the world about my well being. But after I was diagnosed and treated, I refused to follow through with my treatment. It is one thing to come down with health condition; it is another to have a care party working for your return to health.

In my case, I had the best help anyone can wish for. However, I did not take my medication. My refusal caused my health to worsen; I collapsed and placed in ICU more than once!

I need to add that it is not everyone who has the benefit of a second chance. It is therefore essential to remain faithful with the management of CHF once diagnosed. Perhaps, could have the opportunity to breathe fresh air, once more!

Cardiac Arrest

When you survive any health condition reported to have only a 3% survival rate, I bet you need to give thanks to whatever you believe in. As a believer in the miracle-working God, He deserves all praises.

First Anniversary as Cardiac Survivor!

We marked 1st Anniversary of my husband as cardiac arrest survivor on November 01, 2016! If you haven't been through health challenges, you may not appreciate how it feels to survive a chronic illness. However, my experiences watching Richard being through a series of heart-related health crises is better imagined than seen. My husband is a strongman and to see him become so helpless under the grip of chronic illnesses makes me shudder!

Thanks to the Wake County's Emergency Medical Services (EMS) in Raleigh, North Carolina that God used to save my husband. Perhaps without their quick intervention, my husband would have joined the 97% statistics of non-survivors of the terminal health condition. The EMS staff rekindled my confidence in the capacity of our medical services to save lives. Their knowledge and training came in handy in giving Richard second chance at life!

He was revived after his heart stopped for about 40 minutes and all hope for his comeback was lost.

Also, the extraordinary life-saving services provided by Wake County Sheriff's Office, and all of the fire-fighters and police officers from all of our municipalities helped remarkably! Everyone and all agencies are instrumental to the miracle recovery of Richard to which my family is very grateful.

After he left the hospital, following his cardiac arrest and stroke episodes, he was placed on 24-hour care to bring him up to speed in recovery. Thanks to Matt Frazier, Director of the Ruth Sheets Adult Care Center & Staff who weathered the storm with us for many months.

What you should know about the cardiac arrest from the layman's eye

A cardiac arrest survival rate outside a hospital is just six percent, and even when a patient is treated by first responders, it's only 11 percent.

Richard has experienced all the heart conditions with a cheering story to tell as a survivor. My husband was one-time cardiac arrest, two-time heart attack and two –time stroke survivor. He had a heart attack when he was 45 and at 50. At the age of 53, he survived a cardiac arrest and stroke and again he survived a stroke at the age of 56.

While celebrating the first anniversary of his survival, a stranger who thought we were celebrating his birthday offered to take care of the bills. You need to see the joy in his eyes when he learnt it was a thanksgiving for surviving cardiac arrest. His name is John McDonald, and we are grateful for his show of love to rejoice with our family.

A heart attack describes a condition when the flow of blood to the heart is blocked. Cardiac arrest happens when the heart malfunctions due to electrical interruption and suddenly stops beating. As for stroke, it is a brain attack when blood flow to the brain is cut off, leading to brain cell damage.

Medically, cardiac arrest is the sudden loss of heart function in a heart disease patient. It may happen abruptly, or due to other symptoms. If immediate and appropriate steps at recovery aren't taken, cardiac arrest is usually fatal accounting for about 97% loss of life.

First responder and cardiac arrest

During my episodes, I would say I am blessed with a faster response; it is not in every case of cardiac arrest that the patients are so blessed! The first responder during cardiac arrest is crucial to give the patient immediate and urgent attention they deserve to regain consciousness.

Because cardiac arrest relates to an electrical malfunction in the heart that causes an irregular heartbeat, there is a need for immediate medical attention to revive the patient.

Heart sickness could lead to cardiac arrest or stroke. Therefore, it is vital to treat the problem fast when it is discovered.

The chances of having trained the first responder within material time to save a life will depend on how conscious and ready you are as someone living with a heart condition. Medical technologists and scientists have developed various tools and means for early detection of heart crisis.

Tools, such as Wearable cardioverter-defibrillator, can improve survival from cardiac arrest. Also, having adequate knowledge about available help in your environment, such as Wake County EMS and calling 911 would get you immediate medical attention to survive. Early warning signals and adhering to medical advice on care for heart health is essential to your survival.

While you could avoid heart health complications by complying with the Dos and Don'ts after you are diagnosed with a heart condition, heart education is a priority for every family. Heart education prepares the individual to know what to do when the unexpected happened.

Post cardiac arrest and stroke care is a 24-hour call. You need every available medical resource to get the accelerated recovery and pull through it. Unless you are adequately educated about heart health, finding your way in the heat of crises might be a little tight.

More importantly, how soon your first responders are available will determine your survival. The possibility of surviving a Cardiac Arrest decreases by 7-10% at every passing minute without a first responder. This is why defibrillator is recommended as it effectively improves the chances of survival up to 95 percent.

Lesson learned

Although cardiac arrest is a life-threatening heart condition, you can increase your chances of survival with proper education and compliance. Like most people new to hearth heart, I did not follow prescribed medical advice upon diagnosis until I passed out.

From benign high blood pressure, you can degenerate into a life-threatening heart problem if you do not follow medical advice and use your medications. It is glory to God and thanks to the people around me, especially my wife that I could speak as a survivor, many didn't have that privilege!

Importance of Diabetes Self-Management Education

There is no denying the fact that increased prevalence of diabetes in our current society has correspondingly increased the cases of people with diabetes in the hospitals. Diabetes is a severe illness which many of its victims fail to detect at the very onset of it, those who could detect earlier, usually do not take heeds as to how to manage it through proper nutrition and management. This was the case with my husband, when he was diagnosed with type 2 diabetes in 2005.

In 2004, my husband had symptoms of hyperglycemia for some months before diagnosis. He had fasting blood glucose records indicating values of 117-129 mg/dl, which were defined to us as borderlines of diabetes. We both didn't take it seriously as he continued to subsist on his dietary plans; nothing changed from his usual daily intake.

Therefore, we decided that we adhere strictly to medical nutrition therapy to improve his glucose control. Now, I am more knowledgeable about my husband condition so much so that I routinely check his blood sugar level and prepare him, low carb meals all the time.

Furthermore, those specialists made me realize the importance of foot care and my husband's inability presently to feel the light touch of the monofilament. They also charged us to be more vigilant in checking his feet for any possible skin lesions caused by poorly footwear worn when doing exercise.

Lastly, I believe so strongly that self-management education is crucial to managing type 2 diabetes and that, partnership with specialists will reinforce medical nutrition therapies and help improve glucose control in diabetes patients.

Delirium: A Case of Confusion, Agitation, and General Deterioration

Delirium has been described for many years as cardiac manifestations and cognitive disturbance with temporal fluctuation that occur due to rapid changes in the brain function. Though it is temporary and reversible, it is a severe case of mental and physical illness that can never be forgotten in a hurry by those who witnessed it occurring.

There have been several studies about how it does happen. Some schools of thought believe that it occurs due to the inability of the brain to receive enough oxygen or other substance needed in the general cognitive functions. This way, dangerous toxins are accumulated in the brain, and the result is what is called Delirium. This is exactly what we are told at the hospital when my husband had his own share of this not so good experience.

Shortly after the stroke that kept my husband and me at the hospitals for months, Delirium set in. I initially didn't understand what was going on and many thoughts kept contending in my head about what I saw that day as my husband was utterly confused, had difficulties in thinking, remembering and paying attention.

The first thing I noticed was that he looked so devastated and moody. It perceived him thinking those people in the Television are actually with us in the room. It was just in a sorry state and so sad to behold. Initially, I was gravely afraid of him being placed in a mental institution, and within a week, it was gone and normalcy restored.

The same thing happened at the hospital on August 2019. Though he was just being cleared of flash pulmonary edema and within 45 minutes of my arriving at the hospital, the ugly event reared its ugly head again.

During this time, I tried to think of him being apprehensive of those around him generally. He forgot and was totally confused as he thought he was in a hotel, and those around him were trying to rip him off and steal from him. While sleeping with him, he made an escape move and all thanks to the Behavioral Health who was on standby and got a hold of him. He refused his medication as he thought those medicines would complicate his issues and get sicker. However, the management of the hospital was magnanimous enough and gave us certified nurse assistants who sit in the room to him.

I learned a lot during this time as to the importance of good health, and how good health is underappreciated in our current society and you see some people voluntarily giving themselves some issues to deal with in the future. Of course, I was thankful to the sitter while I also stayed with him day and night. When Francisco Diaz who is my husband barber gave him a fresh cut, the Delirium cleared and we joke far more about these events whenever our minds go down the memory lane.

Flash Pulmonary Edema

Sudden scares can seriously jeopardize health! Even if it seems a tad unbelievable, let me narrate a simple incident that occurred in the early hours of 5th August 2019, and you will be convinced! My husband and I heard a loud banging on our front door at 7 am on the day in question. It roused us quickly from sleep – in fact, my husband jumped on his scooter and started pedaling swiftly into the back room. When I got to the door, I spotted a male in the parking lot – he was searching for a suitable spot. On speaking to him, I realized he had mistakenly knocked on our door – he was actually looking for someone who loved across the street.

I went back inside and began to prepare my husband's breakfast, but stopped when I heard him coughing severely. I rushed to the back room and was met with a scary sight – he was on the floor and gasping due to shortness of breath. I called 911 and immediately took him to the hospital where I narrated the entire incident of someone knocking on our door and him taking the scooter to the back room, to the medical staff.

They attended to him and told me that my husband had Flash Pulmonary Edema, which occurs due to the rapid elevation of the left ventricular end-diastolic pressure. Absence of underlying valve disease or cardiomyopathy, it is usually caused by renal vascular disease. It may frequently develop in case of bilateral renal artery stenosis (RAS), unilateral RAS and accompanying functional solitary kidney.

The result was that my husband had to be put on a ventilator for 6 days – it seemed like an eternity! It took 3 tries for the medical staff to get him off the device. The first couple of times when they tried, he became extremely agitated, causing his blood pressure and heart rate to spike dangerously. New medications for the heart were recommended and thankfully it worked, because they were able to get him off the ventilator on the 3rd try. I am very grateful to the efficient medical staff and of course, I never fail to thank the Almighty for seeing us through these tough times.

Stroke

My husband has survived two strokes, so I have first-hand knowledge of how painful and stressful it can be, not only for the person who has suffered through it, but for their family as well.

Heart attack and stroke is often used interchangeably in layman's terms but even though a few symptoms are similar, they are both quite different from each other. A heart attack occurs when blood flow to a part of the heart is blocked, usually by a blood clot. Without oxygenated blood, the heart muscle begins to die. A stroke occurs when the blood supply to the brain is interrupted, which cuts off vital blood flow and oxygen. It happens when a blood vessel feeding the brain gets clogged or bursts.

Take a look at the symptoms of a stroke:

- Face drooping on one side, like a lopsided smile

- Trouble while walking

- Weakness or numbness in an arm or leg, particularly on one side of the body

- Confusion, like you can't think clearly or do something you can normally do

- Slurred speech

- Tongue doesn't work on one side

- Severe & sudden headache

Types of strokes:

Ischemic stroke

It occurs due to a blockage or clot in a blood vessel in your brain. The blockage can be caused when a substance called plaque builds up on the inside wall of an artery.

Hemorrhagic stroke

When a blood vessel in the brain bursts and bleeds, it deprives an area of the brain of blood, which leads to damage. High blood pressure tends to weaken arteries over time, and can lead to this type of stroke. Hemorrhagic stroke is defined by the kind of blood vessel causing the damage. An aneurysm (most common) occurs when an artery or ordinary blood vessel within the brain balloons, weakens, and bursts. In rare cases, an abnormal, tangled mass of blood vessels forms in the brain, which is known as arteriovenous malformation – when one of the vessels within the mass bursts, it leads to bleeding and compression in the brain.

Transient ischemic attack (TIA)

It is also known as a mini or warning stroke and caused by a small clot that briefly blocks an artery. Symptoms generally last less than an hour;

often for just a few minutes. It is a clear indication of a more serious stroke waiting to occur!

It is quite alarming to note that stroke is the 3rd leading cause of death in the United States. Treatment is always most effective when administered within the first few hours after a stroke has occurred, so if you spot any of the symptoms mentioned above, act quickly. If you suspect a stroke, don't delay in calling the EMS – a few minutes' delay could mean the difference between life and death.

Wearable Defibrillator

Back in 2016, my husband was hospitalized due to congestive heart failure. During that time, his left ventricular ejection fraction was 25%, which is shocking to say the least! A normal left ventricular ejection fraction (LVEF) ranges from 55% to 70%. An LVEF of 65%, for example means that 65% of the total amount of blood in the left ventricle is pumped out with each heartbeat.

That is when the doctors suggested a Wearable Cardioverter Defibrillator or WCD. It wasn't a one-stop solution to our problems. In fact, we were pretty apprehensive and shocked. My husband's biggest fear was that the vest will go off and he would fumble when it comes to turning it off. Sometimes the electrode belt would move out of place and generate a loud noise. He had to keep wearing it at night too, while he slept and when he changed positions, it alerted us with sounds. The metal pieces also started bruising his skin.

But even so, the WCD is certainly worth the risk and discomfort for those patients who are at risk for sudden cardiac arrest. It lets doctors monitor the patient's arrhythmic risk closely and take appropriate action. To put it in a nutshell, it detects abnormal heart rhythms and is a form of protection. Despite the initial uneasiness while wearing it, the vest is lightweight and convenient to put on. The vest can easily be worn under your clothing – it contains the electrodes to pick up the patient's electrocardiogram (ECG). The monitor is worn around the waist or from a shoulder strap.

If the WCD detects any life-threatening rapid heart rhythms, it automatically delivers a treatment shock to restore normal heart rhythm. The device alerts a patient right before administering a treatment shock – if the patient is conscious, they can respond to the alarm by pressing the buttons to stop or delay the treatment sequence. If the patient becomes unconscious, the device is designed to release a special gel over the therapy electrodes and deliver an electrical shock to restore normal rhythm.

If the patient's heartbeat returns to normal after the shock is administered, the alarms stop, while the device starts operating in normal monitoring mode once again. But if the arrhythmia continues, the treatment cycle is repeated till 5 treatment cycles are completed. It is advisable to get medical help immediately if the WCD doesn't appear to work!

Music is Good for the Soul
When in the Hospital

When you are down with a chronic illness, one way to get your healing is by listening to soul-moving music. I am familiar with the saying: "music is the language of the soul," but didn't give much thought to it until I saw it in practice with my husband. When all communications seem to breakdown and ineffective, music was able to reach the depth of his soul and gave him strength.

I do know that when your vibration is down and in a state of dormancy, it gives room for pesky diseases in your body. But how can you get your vibration kicking and in motion? One thing common for people battling health problems is being down, psychologically broken!

I have heard and seen my husband cry bitterly and muse aloud the sad statement: "if I would ever walk again!" It's such a spirit dampening musing, which as his wife, sent nerve breaking chill down my spine! But apart from medicine, one thing trained nurses do is how to boost their patient's psychology to overcome negative thoughts.

When you boost a patient's psyche, it accelerates their healing and re-covery. I recall a nurse asking that tune the television to a station that played music for my husband's viewing. Frankly, I didn't see any rele-vance of music to Richard's healing until I started to see how, from his reactions.

There were several songs played, but two are his favourites including "Never Would Have Made It & the Best in me" by Marvin Sapp. As he began to listen to the lyrics, Richard's vibration gradually increased, and his healing accelerated; praise God!

Music Is Awesome For the Mind, Body, and Soul

This claim has the backing of research by authorities in mind healing process. I might not be a psychologist, but I can tell white from black when I see it. Richard's dramatic healing is, partly, thanks to music. It was his impressive recovery that triggered my interest in music as a good recipe for healing the mind, body and soul.

The reasons experts recommend music for everyone, including those living with chronic illness, draw from the following benefits:

- Mood altering powers. Listening to soul-lifting music can change your mood from sadness to happiness. It can boost your vibration to release health producing hormones. When you are happy, your body immunity becomes more potent to fight off diseases and give you health.

- Stress-reducing ability. Stress is everywhere, especially for the sick ones admitted in the hospital for different health problems. When you listen to music, it alleviates your body stressors to give health.

- Boost your self-awareness. Imagine the line from Marvin Sapp music "The Best In Me" that reads:

"… I said he saw the best in me,

When everyone else around

Could only see the worst in me,

(I wish I had a witness tonight, all I need is one)…"

Isn't this soul lifting?

The human brain is wired to carry out the subconscious message delivered to it. The song by Marvin sure touched Richard that his whole being wanted to show the best in him.

I thank God I could be a witness when he saw the best in him as proclaimed by God in that music. Marvin Sapp was, simply, relaying God's message that Richard is not the sick man he thought he was! I saw health in him the way he sees health in himself; praise God!

- It strengthens empathy. When we are sick, it is easy to condemn ourselves to a lifeless body in bed. We tend not to believe anything said by the doctor or relatives about getting well again. If you don't trust medicine, people and all efforts made at regaining health, the battle over sickness is lost! But with soul-lifting music, the table is turned against the illness, and you begin to see yourself as a victor and allow the healer in you take charge!

- Spiritual bonding. Man is foremost a spiritual being. Provided you dwell in the spirit, your entire being will tap from the endless power source of the universe. Think again, why does religion places so much importance on music? It is to serve as a connection between the human and spiritual worlds to make you operate in both planes simultaneously.

For the moment, imagine the connecting power of another line of Richard's favourites of Marvin Sapp music:

"…Never would have made it

Never would have made it without You

I would have lost it all

But now I see how you were there for me…"

It is reassuring of the power of God available in us!

The connecting power of Marvin's "Never Would Have …" music must have been responsible for the remarkable transformation of Richard after a series of admission at the ICU and life support.

Impact of music on the soul

The best way to prove a scientific claim is to see it happen in real life. Richard's dramatic recovery is thanks to medical help we could get and the incredible impact of his favourite gospel songs from Marvin Sapp.

The following are ways music can impact your soul.

Sentimental value

Music has a powerful emotional impact on the listeners; such sentiment is not something you can pick up just anywhere. This sentiment as espoused in his song "the best in me," Marvin says…

"…He saw the best in me,

(When everyone else around me)

When everyone else around (OOOOh)

(Could only see)

Could only see the worst in me,

(Does anybody have that testimony? When folk walks you off, Said you would never make it, what did he see?)…"

The song's lyrics are hard to comprehend for people who are not going through the cliff of life, where hope is lost, and self-believe gives way to doubt about survival.

Romance

Of course, romance and music are inseparable as they enjoy heavenly bond. Music can trigger a romantic feeling to get people in love to connect from the inside. It rekindles the love shared between two people and breaks barriers. The thought of losing a loved one can cause people to fight back with everything in them for self-rescue. Drawing immense energy from within triggered by soul-lifting music helped Richard to bounce back to life with a clutching hold to be with his family.

Healing power

Music is a universal language that is understood by people from all corners of the world, even if rendered in a language not understood. Contained in Richard's favourite songs are powerful healing messages capable of immense miracles. The message, when released, is analysed by the brain to release endorphins to cause great healings.

Motivator

Music benefits the sick by serving as a great motivator to cause them to defy all suggestions of sickness and embrace health. The messages in music can cause you to take your drug as and when due and motivate you to shed unhealthy weight, exercising. There is an endless possibility of achievements under soul music motivation.

When next you feel down or indisposed, I urge you not to be depressed, get up find good soul lifting music and listen. If you can, get up and dance away your sorrow because music helps to boost your spirit!

Signs of Heart Attacks to Watch Out For- Always Be Alert!

At times you don't think that a terrible incident you read or heard about can happen to you or your loved ones, till it actually does and frightens the hell out of you. A similar instance occurred in my life when my husband had not one but two heart attacks in 2008 and 2013.

How it happened?

On the day of the first attack in 2008, he was complaining about not feeling like himself, and wanted to stay home and rest. Only when he began to experience pain in his chest, did we go to a hospital. I had given him an aspirin as suggested by a past co-worker, who told me to do so if I ever got the indications that my husband was having a heart attack. The doctor thoroughly examined him and was almost prepared to let him go but he ordered some additional tests to be on the safe side. When the reports arrived, the doctor asked if my husband was administered an aspirin at home. When I said yes, he told me that my husband had suffered a slight heart attack, so he had to be admitted.

His 2nd heart attack in 2013 was much worse as he had to be put on life support due to congestive heart failure. It was a long road to recovery with intense physical therapy and medication, and there was yet another rocky patch in 2015 when he had a stroke and went into cardiac arrest. However, he survived and came out much stronger from the ordeal – rather we both did!

Signs of heart attack

That is why I urge you to stay alert for possible signs of heart attacks – tragedy strikes without warning; it could happen to you or someone close like a friend or family member. Here are some common signs to watch out for:

- Acute chest pain or discomfort

- Nauseous feeling

- Excessive sweating

- Light-headedness or dizziness

- Fatigue

Tips to prevent heart disease

Apart from the ones mentioned above, there are other symptoms that might occur, or there might be no manifestation of any discomfort but you could have a heart attack. Prevention is better than cure as they say, so I have compiled a list of tips that can help prevent heart diseases, which is increasing at an alarming rate with every year.

- High blood pressure is a major risk, so get your blood pressure checked regularly – at least once a year for adults, and more often if you have high blood pressure.

- Keep cholesterol and triglyceride levels in check or they clog arteries and boost risk of coronary artery disease and heart attack.

- Maintain a healthy body weight as being overweight can contribute to heart disease.

- Try to limit saturated fats, foods high in sodium, and added sugars. Eat plenty of fresh fruits, vegetables, and whole grains.

- Create fitness routine and stick to it – proper exercise strengthens your heart and improves circulation.

- Limit alcohol if you can't quit entirely – it raises blood pressure and causes weight gain, which in turn leads to heart disease.

- Cigarette smoking raises your blood pressure and puts you at higher risk for heart attack and stroke, so if you are a smoker, you have to steer clear gradually.

Unfortunately, there is no guarantee or sure-shot method of preventing heart attacks and related disease. We can only lead a healthy lifestyle, stay alert, and hope for the best!

Managing Heart Health:
What you eat matters

While it is essential to discuss heart health and how you can overcome any heart condition, it is imperative to talk about what you eat. It is not a joke the saying "you are what you eat," and if you want to get well or avoid getting sick, it's high time you started watching your food.

You may be a lover of a particular food because of its health benefits, but your healthy food changed the moment it is cooked. In the cook's efforts to achieve tasty food, sodium and other ingredients are added. A simple culinary education teaches that cooking changes the state of the food you cook and what is added can make the meal toxic in your body.

Let me tell you a story…

I do not buy salt, and I have not cooked with it in over 20 years. However, I understand that the health nutrition buzzword – low sodium diet, means more than not cooking with salt. You should be careful how you apply your knowledge of a low sodium diet because it's everywhere!

Yes, the majority of the food we buy at the eateries and food canteens are loaded with salt. I don't mean to spoil any food business. My point is that we should start to care about the quantity of salt we consume.

Despite my conscious avoidance of the use of salt in my food for over 20 years, my husband still suffered stroke and CHF.

The majority of the foods we buy have a disturbing quantity of salt. My husband is on a 1500 mg low sodium diet. I have to read food labels. I cook with Mrs. Dash, Garlic Powder, Trader Joe's 21 Seasoning, lemon, Vinegar, Basil and minced garlic. It has been trying hard to make his food tasty and keep foods low sodium.

Not many of us are aware of the danger of consuming salt, called sodium, in excess. For the love of tasty food, we often binge on a particular food, thereby consuming more sodium than is appropriate. The result is a gradual deterioration of our body organs like kidney, liver with consequences for aggravating diabetic tendency in our body system.

Therefore, eating healthy is not limited to fresh food only; the way you cook is also of utmost importance.

If you desire to eat healthy, which I think you should, it's time to learn as a matter of urgency the following nutrition buzzwords:

Low Sodium Diet

Consuming a low sodium diet is a recommended way to manage heart failure. Sodium is a mineral in many foods with salt as the chief custodian. It means salt is not the only food item with sodium, but the quantity of sodium in salt is way too high to consume too much of it.

The effect of salt in the body is water retention; it causes the body to retain too much water, which also affects the heart. Therefore, maintaining a low sodium diet helps to keep high blood pressure and edema condition (swelling) under control.

It is essential to know that sodium content in every food varies per serving. You should talk to your doctor to know the tolerable sodium intake for you and try to stay within the threshold now to avoid being sorry later.

Low Carb Diet

Every class of food has its purpose in the body. Dietary experts have facts about what each food type supplies in the overall nutritional contribution to the body. With this knowledge, certain foods have been restricted while others are tolerable for consumption.

Since carbs have been identified as contributing to weight gain, which in the long run, affects your heart health, food experts recommend a low-carb diet for weight-loss.

If you are managing heart condition or you plan to avoid slipping into heart problems, it is essential to consider a low carb diet. There is a long list of foods to avoid, but chief among them include Sugar, Refined Grains, Trans fats, low-fat products, processed foods, among others.

Low-carb foods include Meat, Fish, Eggs, Vegetables, Nuts and seeds, Fruits, Fats and oils and high-fat dairy.

You may think because you are healthy, you have a license for carefree nutrition; this is the wrong way to think. You should know that what you become tomorrow is a result of what you do today. Since we are what we eat, what will you become in 5, 10 or 15 years from now?

With adherence to low sodium and low carb diets, your job at having the perfect meal isn't complete until you consider how you cook your food. Here, the way you cook your meal says a lot about how healthy your food will become. For this reason, I will share my experiences using Air Fryer and Instant Pot Pressure Cooker.

Air Fryer

This product provides an efficient and hassle-free way to cook your food such as chicken wings, boneless chicken breast, fries, and so many other food items. There are different brands of Air Fryer you can get in the market. Having such an excellent cooking tool helps to achieve the right energy release for cooking outstanding food.

Instant Pot Pressure Cooker

I wasn't a lover of the pressure cooker until I realized the benefits it has in the kitchen. As a versatile kitchen appliance, it offers consistent great results in the food you prepared for wholesome health. You don't have a problem in determining the temperature to cook with and timing the duration your food stays on the heat.

Among several benefits you will get using Instant Pot Pressure Cooker include time and energy saving, food nutrient retention. You know certain nutrients like vitamins and minerals get lost in the cause of cooking due to excess heat. Losing such nutritional value in your food is a waste of money as you get less dietary worth from your meal.

I also found that a pressure cooker can help to preserve the inviting appearance of your food as well as the aroma! Cooking your food at the right temperature and timing helps to eliminate harmful microorganisms and give you wholesome health!

Let me conclude by admonishing you to take extra care of your food.

Life is too precious to careless about what you eat because in the end; you are what you eat!

Ejection Infraction

What is ejection fraction?

Ejection fraction is actually a measurement of the percentage of blood that leaves your heart every time it contracts. The heart functions by contracting and relaxing – when it contracts, blood is ejected from the two pumping chambers (ventricles) and when your heart relaxes, the ventricles refill with blood. Regardless of the force of the contraction, the heart is unable to pump all the blood out of the ventricle. This is where the term "ejection fraction" comes into play – it refers to the percentage of blood pumped out of a filled ventricle with each heartbeat.

How is reduced ejection fraction caused?

There are numerous factors that can contribute to reduced ejection fraction, such as:

o   Weakness of the heart muscle, such as cardiomyopathy.

o   Heart attack that damaged the heart muscle.

o   Heart valve problems.

o   Long-term, uncontrolled high blood pressure.

What is normal ejection fraction?

This is one of the many tests your doctor uses to determine how your heart works and if it is functioning as it should be. But even with a normal ejection fraction, your overall heart function may not be normal. After my husband has a cardiac arrest in November, 2015, his ejection fraction was 25. It improved slightly in the next few months and went up between 35 and 40. He was stable till August, 2019, but after we had an incident of a man knocking on the wrong door, which caused heart problems yet again, his ejection fraction was back to 25. The doctors are now saying he is in his last stage of congestive heart failure.

The ejection fraction is usually measured only in the left ventricle (LV). The left ventricle is the heart's main pumping chamber. It pumps oxygen-rich blood up into the upward (ascending) aorta to the rest of the body.

- o An LV ejection fraction of 55 percent or higher is considered normal.

- o An LV ejection fraction of 50 percent or lower is considered reduced.

- o An LV ejection fraction between 50 and 55 percent is usually considered "borderline."

Transesophageal Echocardiogram (TEE)

What is a transesophageal echocardiogram (TEE)?

It is a special type of echocardiogram that is usually done when the doctor wishes to look more closely at your heart to determine if it could be producing blood clots. Like an echocardiogram, the TEE uses high-frequency sound waves (ultrasound) to examine the structures of the heart. A transducer is used for directing sound waves – it is placed in the esophagus that connects the mouth to the stomach, and since it is close to the heart, images from a TEE gives clear images of the heart and its surrounding structures.

What can you expect?

You could be given a mild sedative that helps to relax. During the procedure, it is normal to administer oxygen. The throat is numbed using an anesthetic, while a flexible tube about the size of your index finger is inserted into the mouth and down the esophagus. During the procedure, you may feel the probe moving, but it generally isn't painful nor does it interfere with your breathing. The transducer at the tip of the tube releases sound waves that bounce off your heart and are converted into pictures on a video screen. The doctor can move the tube up, down and sideways to look at different parts of your heart from different angles. The test usually takes about 20 to 40 minutes.

What happened to my husband…a word of caution!

After my husband had a stroke in August 2018, the cardiologist recommended a TEE test. Right before the test, I had told the doctor that I changed my mind about my husband taking the TEE test as I had concerns regarding the anesthesia being administered to him. The doctor was surprised and kept asking me whether I didn't want to know what his numbers are. I was scared, but gave the green light for the test. I sat in the waiting room alone and prayed for everything to be alright.

After the test, my husband said his throat hurt and he wasn't able to eat anything. The nurse consulted the doctor and gave him throat lozenges, but to no avail, because his throat continued to hurt. I informed the nurse that he wasn't getting any relief. Hours later, a test was conducted to find out what the problem was; it turned out his throat was closing up as the doctor had hit the esophagus during the TEE. It had a tear due to which my husband was suffering. There is a 1% chance of this occurring, but even so it did happen to us. He was put on a ventilator for a couple of weeks, but he survived! So please make sure you understand the risks before proceeding.

Know Your Numbers

What are the five key numbers?

According to the American Heart Association, it is imperative to be aware about the five important numbers - Total Cholesterol, HDL (good) Cholesterol, Blood Pressure, Blood Sugar and Body Mass Index (BMI).

Why are these numbers crucial?

It is vital that you know about these numbers as it lets your healthcare provider or doctor to understand if you are at risk for developing cardiovascular disease due to atherosclerosis. It includes conditions like angina or chest pain, heart attack, stroke due to blood clots, and Peripheral Artery Disease (PAD).

Your heart health is of the utmost importance!

How can you manage something that hasn't been measured? You must know exactly at what risk you are, in order to prevent cardiovascular disease in future and knowing these numbers is the very first step towards it. Talk to your doctor immediately without further delay as your heart health is dependant on it. My employer takes health insurance very seriously, and makes it compulsory to get our Blood Pressure,

Cholesterol, Blood Sugar and Body Mass Index (BMI) checked regularly every year, so we can assess the risk of heart disease and stroke. In case we don't get the tests, a monthly fee is charged!

Making Your Wish Known

We don't really understand the importance of advance care directives when we are happy and healthy. But disaster strikes without warning, so advance care planning is a must, so you don't feel helpless or distressed when the time arrives.

It happened to me…

Let me tell you my story so you get to know more about advance care directives. It started with my husband's cardiac arrest some years back. While he was in the hospital, he had a stroke as well. It was too much for his body, so after the stroke his vital organs couldn't perform bodily functions without any support. It was imperative that he undergoes life-sustaining treatments to keep him alive and ensure his organs start working properly.

What next?

I spoke to the Palliative Care department and they gave me the option to "pull the plug", if I so wished. It was because my husband had entered a vegetative state so he would never walk, talk, or understand anything. After pondering for a while, I called my family to tell them what was going on. Some time later, I ran into the same doctor who had treated my husband a couple of months back for stomach issues. I spoke to him, explained the current situation, and asked for advice about pulling the plug. He told me not to make hasty decisions, and that it was too soon to consider that option.

How life-sustaining treatments can help?

Speaking to the doctor gave me some hope, so I decided not to pull the plug, and instructed the medical staff to begin life-sustaining treatments. I was in for a pleasant surprise that night as my husband asked for me, and I reassured him that I was right beside him in his hour of need. I ensured that he receives all the life-sustaining treatments listed on the advance health care directive form that we had filled out. Basically, these treatments involve the usage of machines and other equipment to ensure that bodily functions are carried on as usual – take a look:

- Ventilator – a machine that helps to breathe normally.

- Dialysis – a setup that carries out the function of kidneys by eliminating waste from the body.

- Nasogastric Or Gastrostomy Tube – it is inserted into the stomach to provide food.

- Intravenous Tube – it is inserted into the veins to supply fluids and medicines.

- Oxygen Mask – a device for supplying plenty of oxygen to the patient for better breathing.

The crucial aspect is to fill out advance care directives beforehand, so your loved ones know exactly what to do!

Know More about Advance Care Planning

The future is uncertain, so there could be a time when you are unable to make coherent decisions regarding health care. That is why advance care planning is a must to prepare for times when you can't speak for yourself.

What is advance care planning?

Remember, that these decisions are influenced based on your personal values, preferences, and discussions with your loved ones. Advance care planning involves detailed research to find out information regarding the types of life-sustaining treatments currently available, and then deciding what treatment you would opt for, if you are diagnosed with a life-limiting illness. A significant aspect is to complete advance directives like living will and Power of Attorney – whatever you want or don't want, and who should speak on your behalf (when you are unable), needs to be put into writing.

What is a living will?

As mentioned, a living will is an advanced directive, which is a legal document, detailing the type of care an individual wants (or doesn't want), in the event they are unable to communicate their wishes. Doctors and hospitals often consult the living will when a person who suffers from a terminal illness or a life-threatening injury, is unconscious. This is done to determine if the patient wants life-sustaining treatment, such as assisted breathing or tube feeding. A living will has to meet state requirements regarding notarization or witnesses – it is a must if the will is to be considered valid. The document can take effect as soon as it is signed, or only when it is determined that the person can no longer communicate their wishes about treatment.

What is Power of Attorney for health care?

The Durable Power of Attorney (DPOA) is often used with a living will when it comes to health care. At times, the two documents are combined into one. The DPOA basically appoints the person who will carry out wishes regarding end-of-life treatments that are written down in a living will or medical directive.

What Is a MOST form?

This is a doctor's order that lets you remain in control over medical care at the end of life. Medical Orders for Scope of Treatment (MOST) is a new kind of health care directive in North Carolina, which is like a Do Not Resuscitate (DNR) order – it informs emergency medical personnel and other health care providers if they can (or can't) resort to cardiopulmonary resuscitation (CPR) in the event of a medical emergency. Other information about wishes for end-of-life health care can also be mentioned in the MOST form.

Advance care planning is vital in today's times, so if you haven't begun the process, do it ASAP!

Health Care Advocate

I've been serving as my husband advocate for a long time. Prior to this time, I didn't know what to call what I was doing until I spoke with some medical professionals, who used to tell me "you are a good health advocate for your husband." I have also heard a doctor tell him the same too, "your wife is a good health advocate for you."

Isn't that interesting? I ask questions, write down the information, and speak up for him so he can better understand his illness and get the care and resources he needs - giving him a peace of mind so he can focus on his recovery.

This is not limited to my husband. I also serve as my mother's advocate anytime she needs my support. I suppose you also have loved ones, and I would like to advise you to also serve as their health care advocate when needed.

The role of health care advocate ranges from one level to another. Just as parents are expected to take their children's health a priority, some folks within the communities have taken it as their sole responsibilities to check on the healthiness of their neighbors, members of the society, etc. This set of people collaborate with other health care providers to ensure people get proper health care.

Health care advocate serves as health educators, care managers, patient navigators, health advisers, etc. working within medical environments, like hospitals, community health centers, long term care facilities, patient services programs of non-profit organizations, etc.

People like these can also be call patient advocates, though patient advocate work specifically within medical environments working as voluntary health advocates for sick people, especially in a disease dominate environment. However, we all must hold people's health as one of our priorities, thus be a good health advocate for everyone.

Advance Directive Documents for Terminal Illness

Life is precious, and that goes with everything you do in your lifetime. The law secures your right to Life and Own property, and that is binding even if you are unable to talk. The law respects your wishes and privacy as long as you are within the ambit of the law.

It is edifying to know your rights are protected. However, think of the time when your decision is needed in critical times when unable to decide. If, at such time, a crucial decision is required to save your life and you are mentally incapacitated; it can become difficult for your caregiver to proceed.

My experience in this regard was when my husband was critically ill. He could not talk, and a decision about what to do with him almost stalled necessary medical help for him.

Every time Richard was admitted to the hospital, they often asked for an Advance Care Directive. Sometimes they asked if he Code, do you want us to resuscitate him. Code is a medical term for a patient with no heartbeat or breathing.

Richard has had Code situations that he was resuscitated several times. He had a cardiac arrest in 2015 and took the EMS (emergency medical services) 45 minutes to bring him back. And when he got to the hospital, they had to resuscitate him again.

After the third cardiac arrest, he had a stroke 11 days later. When he had his first stroke, I was told by the Palliative Care Personnel that I could pull the plugs. In the judgement of the neurologist, my husband would never walk, talk or comprehend again. It was a high point of my making a life and death decision for Richard.

I had to decide whether to pull the plug and end everything or ask them to proceed and give him everything available for his survival. It was a crossroads for me; pull or not to pull? It was difficult for me because I did not know what my husband would want. He couldn't talk or feel my worries; he was just there with his life in my hands!

Knowing Richard to be a strong and energetic man, he would never choose to be in bed like a vegetable!

As I was thinking and utterly empty of ideas, I was in the hallway looking out the window when my husband Gastroenterologist (GI) came to the rescue. His word of advice was soothing; it gave me a direction on what to do. After I told him my dilemma about pulling the plug; he said it was too soon to call. He said to allow time before such a far-reaching decision is made.

I took the leap of faith and followed the GI's advice; I told the medical staff I was not going to pull the plug and asked them to move forward with treatment. There and then, they swung into action with everything they got on advance care directive. Today, Richard lives and happy; I am joyful too!

You should know that it is the job of the Emergency medical services (EMS) personnel to resuscitate a patient in Code. The only condition they won't perform this task is with a qualified DNR order. However, a valid DNR order issued by a licensed health care facility is not acceptable by EMS personnel outside of the facility.

What is a DNR Order?

It's a medical order, issued by a doctor, instructing health care personnel Do-Not-Resuscitate when a patient's heart stops to beat.

Consider having these documents while you are hale and hearty. You deserve a second chance at life. It will help your caregivers follow your wishes when you are mentally incapacitated.

Let's discuss some of the essential documents you need to have ready just in case:

What is an Advance Directive?

When you are managing terminal illness, you expect there could be a time when you are unable to decide due to various reasons. At such times, it puts your caregiver in a dilemma on what to do regarding your treatment.

If you recall my situation when my husband had a stroke, I had an issue making the call to pull or not to pull the plug. There are times when a patient would collapse and become unresponsive; at such times, they can't decide on their care.

Therefore, advance directives are documents that communicate the patients' preference for health care when they are unable to decide for themselves. These documents will contain the wishes of the patient in writing instructing on what line of action to take regarding their care or property or any decision whatsoever needing their attention.

With advance directives, the patient is helping to resolve possible conflicts as a result of deciding the next line of action during and after his care when he is unable to make a decision himself.

Types of advance directives

Two types of advance directives exist:

1. A living will that communicates types of medical treatment preferred by the patient at the end of life should they be unable to speak or make such call during your treatment;

2. Power of attorney appointing someone you trust makes health care decisions on your behalf in the event you are unable to make such a call. This person so empowered will have far-reaching authority to act on your behalf with regards to life-prolonging health care decisions. This agent becomes your proxy in matters relating to your medical treatments, as stipulated in the document in the event you are unable to communicate your intentions.

The validity of the Advance Directive document

Note, however, that the Advance Directive document has three components parts; these are parts one, two and three. You will have the option to complete parts one and two. But part three is mandatory as it contains your signature, witnessed by two other persons.

I have attached North Carolina **Planning for Important Health Care Decisions** as a sample. The document is published with the permission of the copyright owner. The paper is peculiar to North Carolina, as you will find one for your state if you live in the US.

Also, note that creating an Advance Directive document is something you can draw out yourself without an attorney. Follow the provisions of each section and conclude with signing in the presence of one or more witnesses.

After you have filled the document, make copies for your health care agent and physician. Also, register it with relevant authorities as you will find out more in the North Carolina attached sample.

Advance Care Planning

I love the saying - "Fail to plan is plan to fail," this is more apt for the end of life health management. Before you can arrive at a useful Advance Directive document, you need to get your hand firmly around salient decisions in the document. This is where Advance Care Planning comes into the picture.

You need to understand that Advance Directives contain your decisions about what happened in your end of life treatments. Whoever administers your right to decide in your absence is representing you in every respect. The choices he makes on your behalf is binding. Therefore you need to think it through properly while you are hale and hearty and in the right frame of mind. This is the opportunity you have in Advance Care Planning to ensure the right decision is made!

Hence, advance care planning encompasses the following:

- Find information on available types of life-sustaining treatments

- Decide the types of treatment you would or would not want in the event of a life-limiting illness

- Discussing your principles and preferences with your loved ones

- Complete Advance Directives to commit into writing your preferred and otherwise types of treatment in the event you are mentally incapacitated to speak for yourself

- Consider and decide on the person(s) to speak for you if you are unable to speak for yourself

Sometimes in life, we want to learn vital lessons from others and not be the guinea pig ourselves. There are procedures to make life easier during terminal illness management. But many loved ones have been put in terrible conditions for lack of clear instructions about the wish of a beloved being treated for chronic illness.

Estate Planning Checklist

We all need to think ahead and make provisions of some degree in respect of Estate Planning. End of Life Advance Directive regarding estate Planning deals with organizing personal and financial matters. This document is necessary to make your wishes known, in the event you are not able to deal with it due to mental incapacity or death!

Therefore, to plan your estate when you are hale and hearty, there is a list of actions to take. Although you could develop your estate plan with the help of your attorney, it is essential to have an idea of things to discuss.

The following checklist contains the necessary items to create a sound Estate Planning document that takes care of your wishes.

1. **Cover Estate Planning Basics.** This part takes care of what happens in the event of disability or death. Part of the things to consider include how to deal with your property, your family welfare. It should protect your survivors against any unforeseen adversities and taxation. Notable in this consideration is the guardianship of your minor children, if any, including their medical care.

2. **Plan Asset Ownership.** Your properties, including motor vehicles, real estate, and other assets, come under this checklist. Upon your demise, the document state how ownership and titles are transferred to the beneficiaries without any trouble whatsoever.

3. **Beneficiary Designations.** Designate what of your assets belong to a beneficiary upon your death. While you are alive, the person so designated will not have an ownership right until death comes. Assets best suited for this include bank and other financial accounts, often called pay-on-death, aka POD. Apart from financial or bank assets, other assets such as cars, real estate and life insurance are qualified for Beneficiary Designation.

4. **Cover debts with Insurance.** This is a provision where any debt you owe is provided for by insurance cover. It is to protect your loved ones from being hounded by your creditors upon your disability or death.

5. **Last will or testament done.** This document takes care of any property to be probated. Also, it takes care of any other relevant matters, including taking responsibility for your loved

ones with a disability. It also helps to name your estate executor or appoint a trusted person as a guardian for your minor or disabled kids.

6. **A Living Trust**. Having a Living Trust protect those you are living behind from imminent troubles. This process handles your properties as though you are living and still the one making the calls. A living trust saves your beneficiaries from crises; it avoids probate and minimizes estate taxes.

7. **A Financial Power of Attorney**. The document gives authority to a trusted person to act for you in financial matters. POA, if rightly worded, can become active immediately or at a stipulated event such as when you are mentally incapacitated or at death.

8. **A Health Power of Attorney**. This authorizes a trusted person to act in your health matters upon your mental incapacity and inability to make decisions.

9. **A Living Will.** It is another name for Advance Directive. It states your wishes regarding the type of life-prolonging medical care you like or dislike at a time you are terminally ill and unable to communicate what you want. This document goes with a healthcare power of attorney to guide your appointed agent on what to do in certain health matters.

10. **Leave Information for Executor and Statement of Desires.** Last but not least, is the document stating your desire to the appointed executor. It provides extra guidance and clarifications to your designated agent on how to proceed in the execution of your wishes.

The document helps the people you entrusted with valuable deci-sion-making about your life when you are not able to make decisions to find their way and proceed without a hiccup!

You see, you may already be familiar with these documents or any of it, but they are essential items to have when dealing with a terminal illness. It helps your caregivers to make quick and relevant decisions, just as you would do if you are available.

About The Author

Richard is a strong and healthy man by all standards. After graduating high school, he decided to pursue a career as an entrepreneur running a home-based lawn care and hauling service. As a young man, his lifestyle was typical of what healthy guys in his shoe would do; carefree and larger than life!

However, in late 1997, Mr. Tucker was diagnosed with high blood pressure. There and then, at the ER, he was prescribed medicine for the health condition. Unknown to him the gravity of his health condition, he was less faithful to the prescription. Consequently, his health became worsened with cold and flu. On Valentine's Day, 1998, he suffered another attack requiring Emergency Response, where he was diagnosed with congestive heart failure (CHF).

From 1998 to date, Richard has had been admitted more than 10 times for CHF. He has suffered other chronic health conditions, including H-pylori (stomach ulcers) and pancreatitis. Richard was on ICU on several occasions and life support severally since 1998. In 2018, he suffered a stroke and another medical emergency called pulmonary edema in 2019.

It is rare for one man to go through such a spirit-breaking health condition to survive it. But by the stroke of providence and loving care and untiring caring spirit of his wife and caregivers, Mr. Tucker is alive, a testimony worth hearing. He is a native of Washington, North Carolina, but for the past 33 years of his life resided in Raleigh, North Carolina.

Walking Miracle Photo Gallery

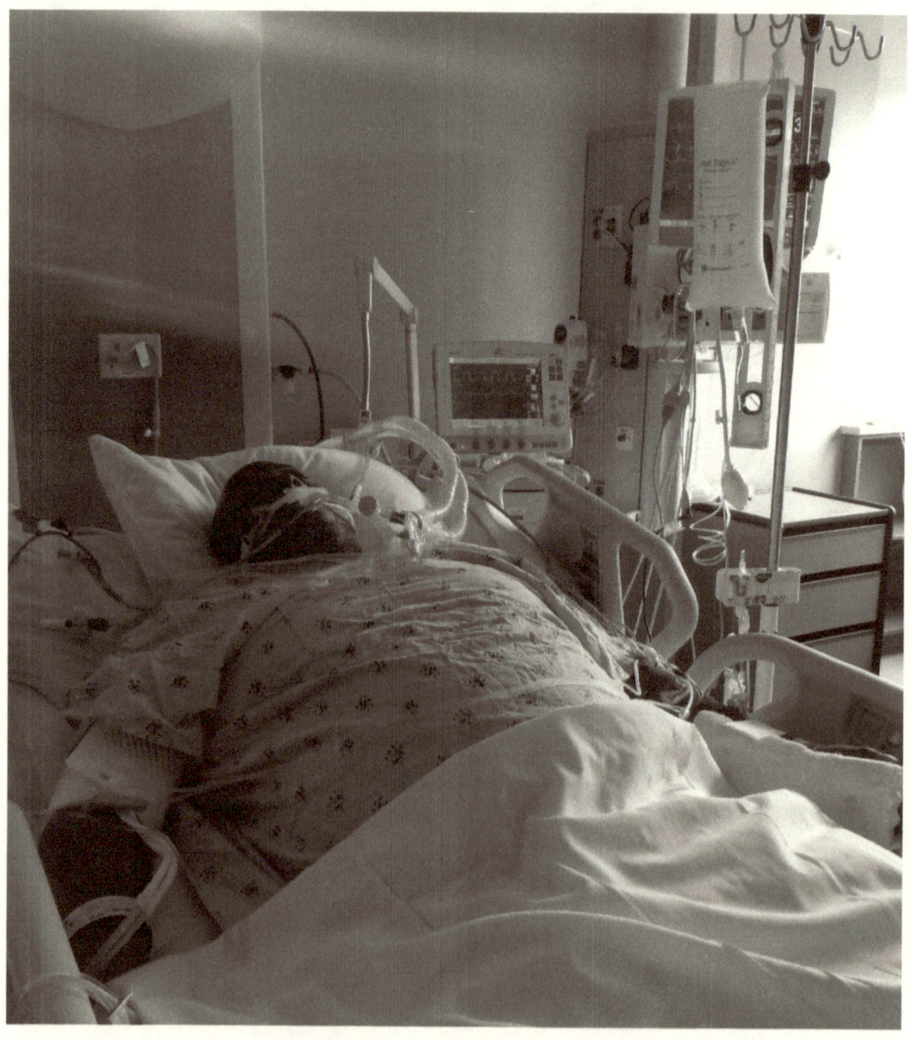

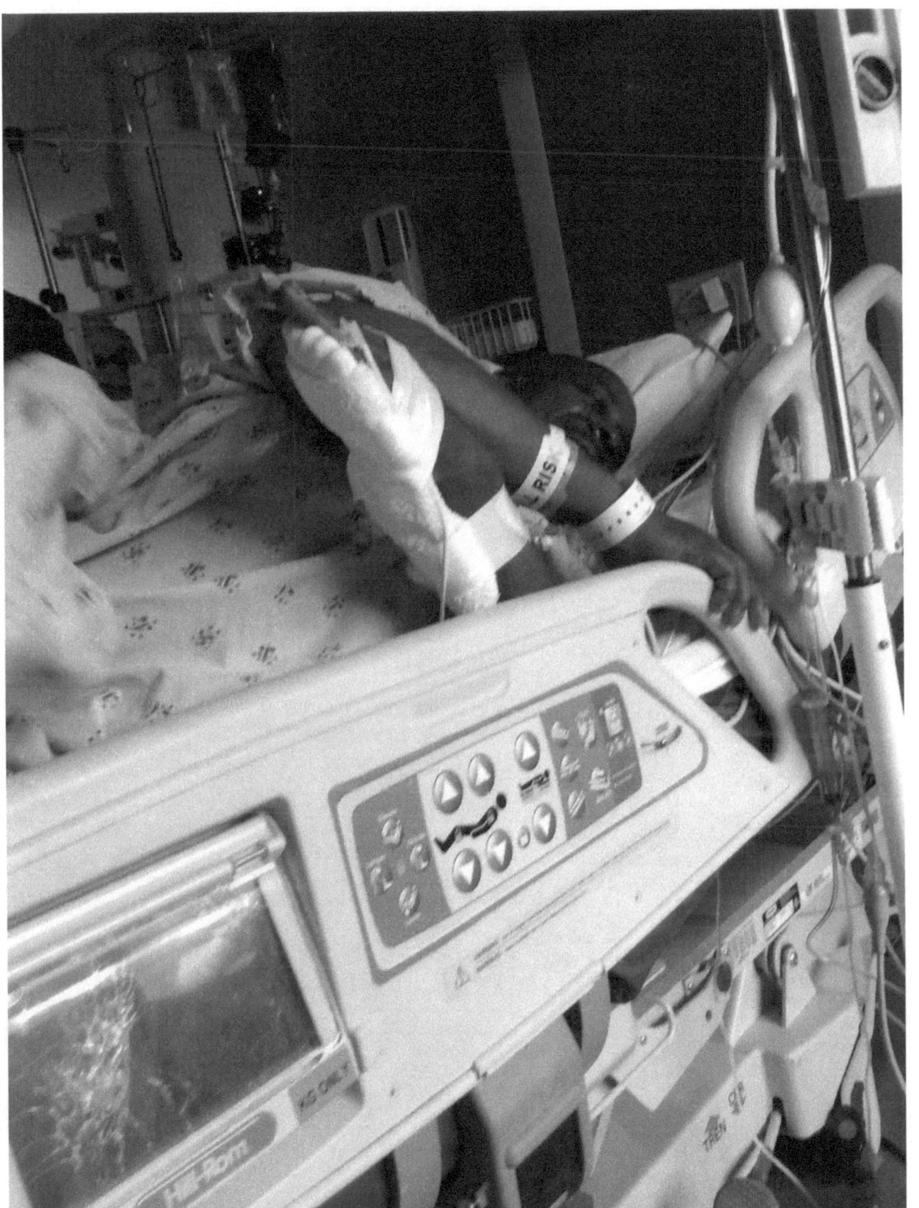

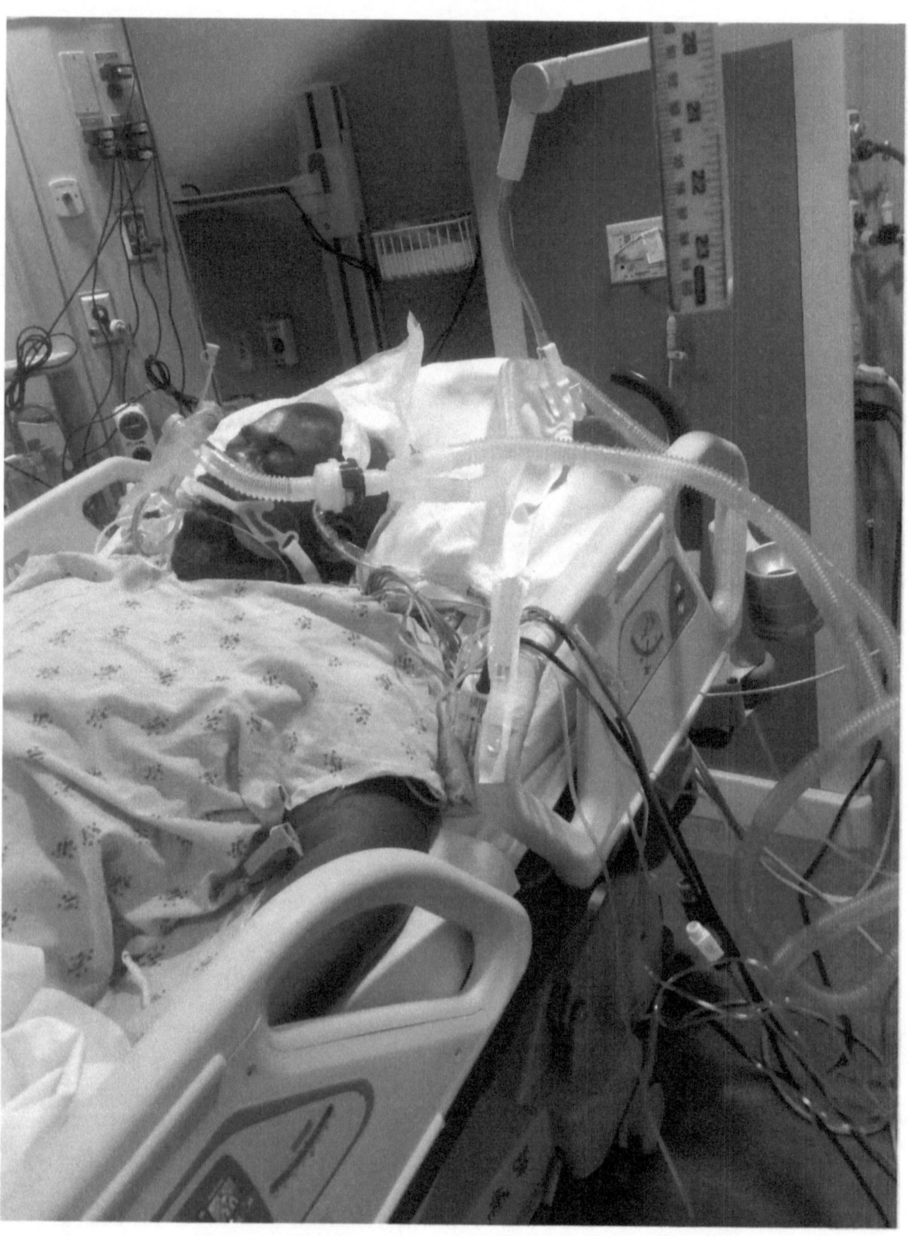

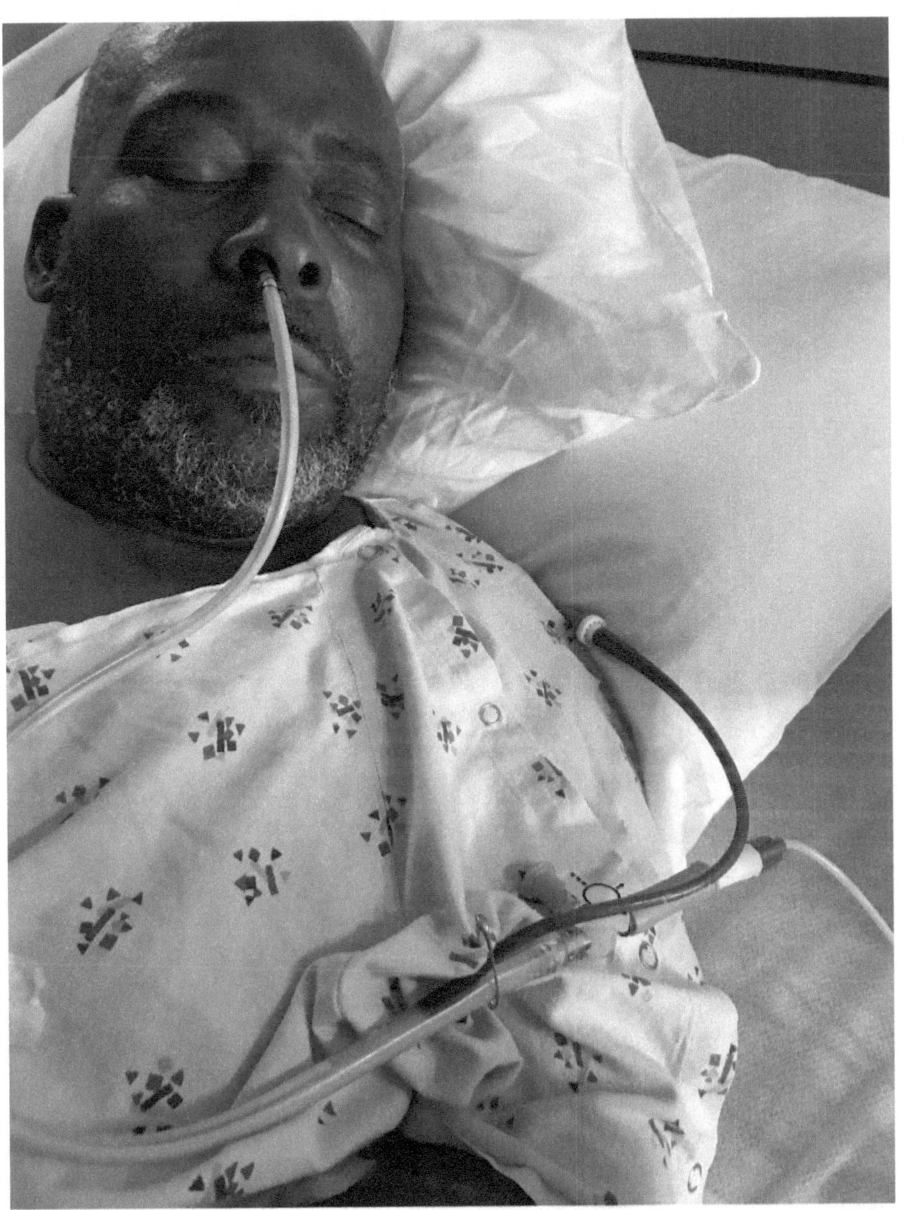

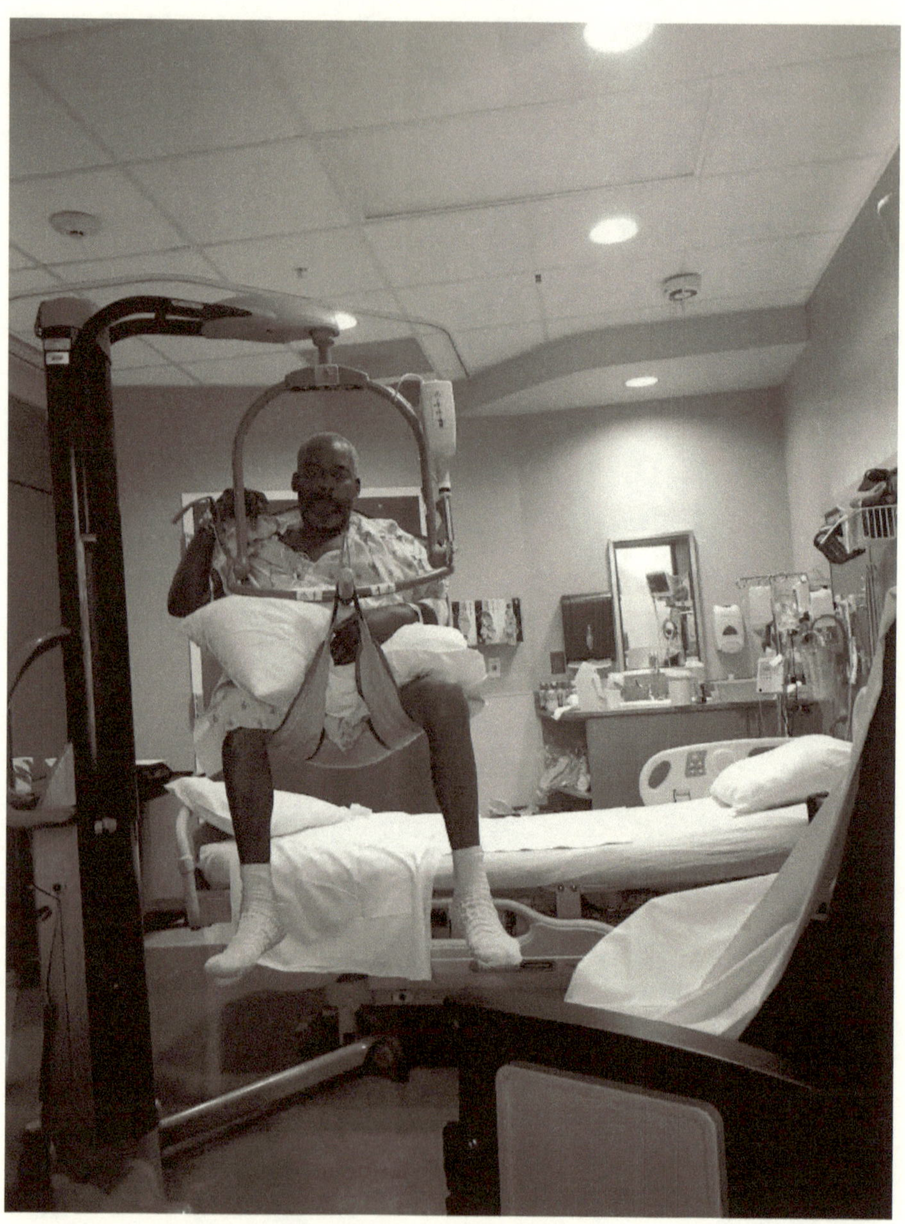

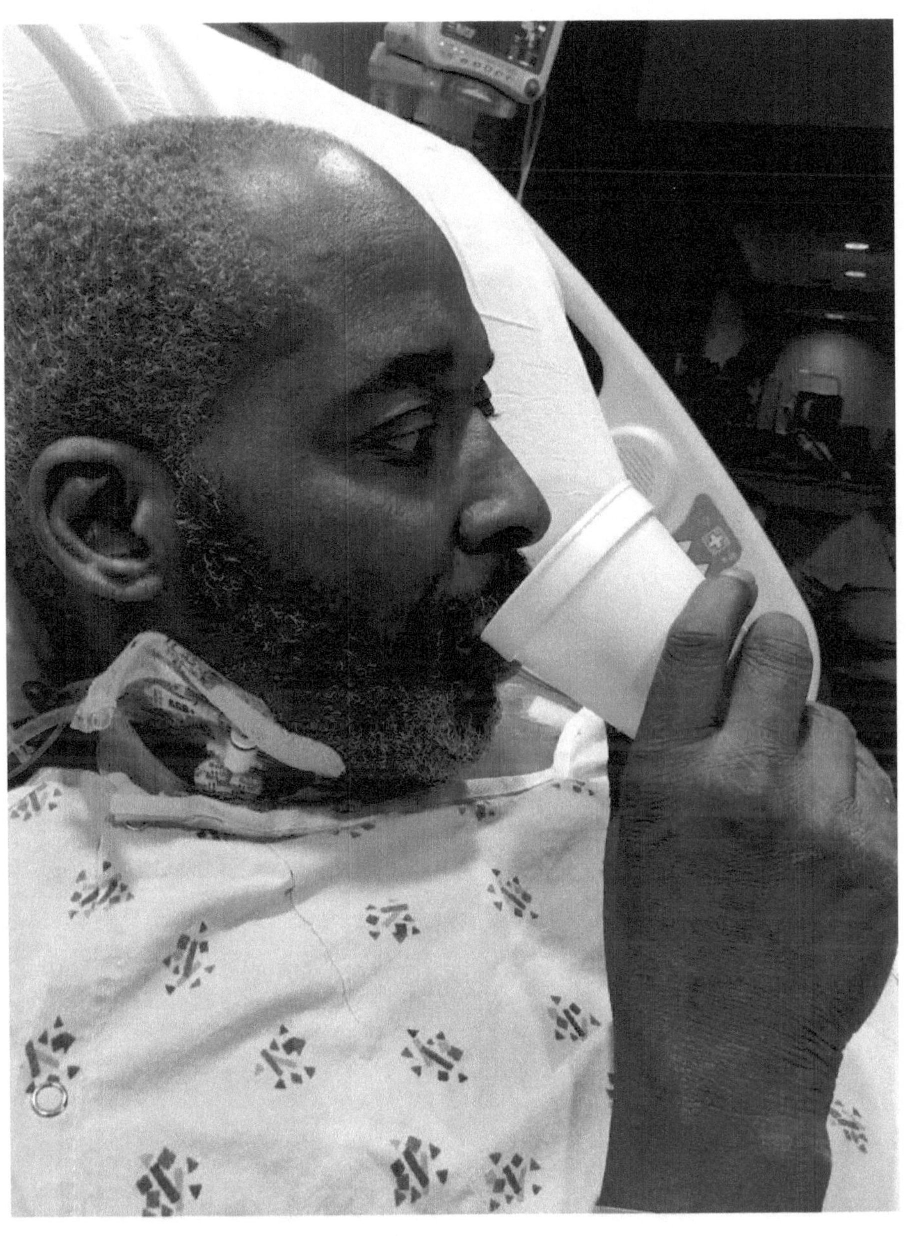

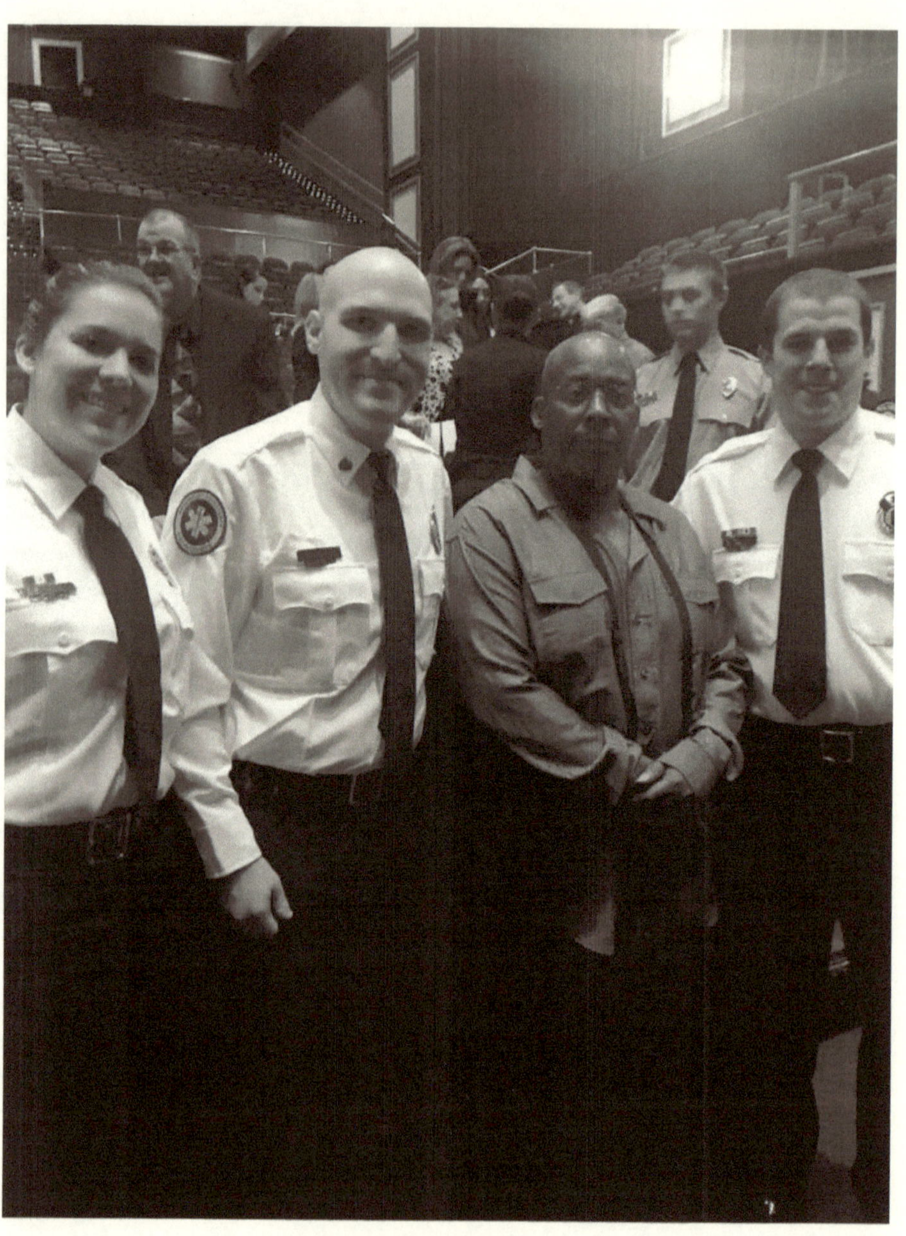

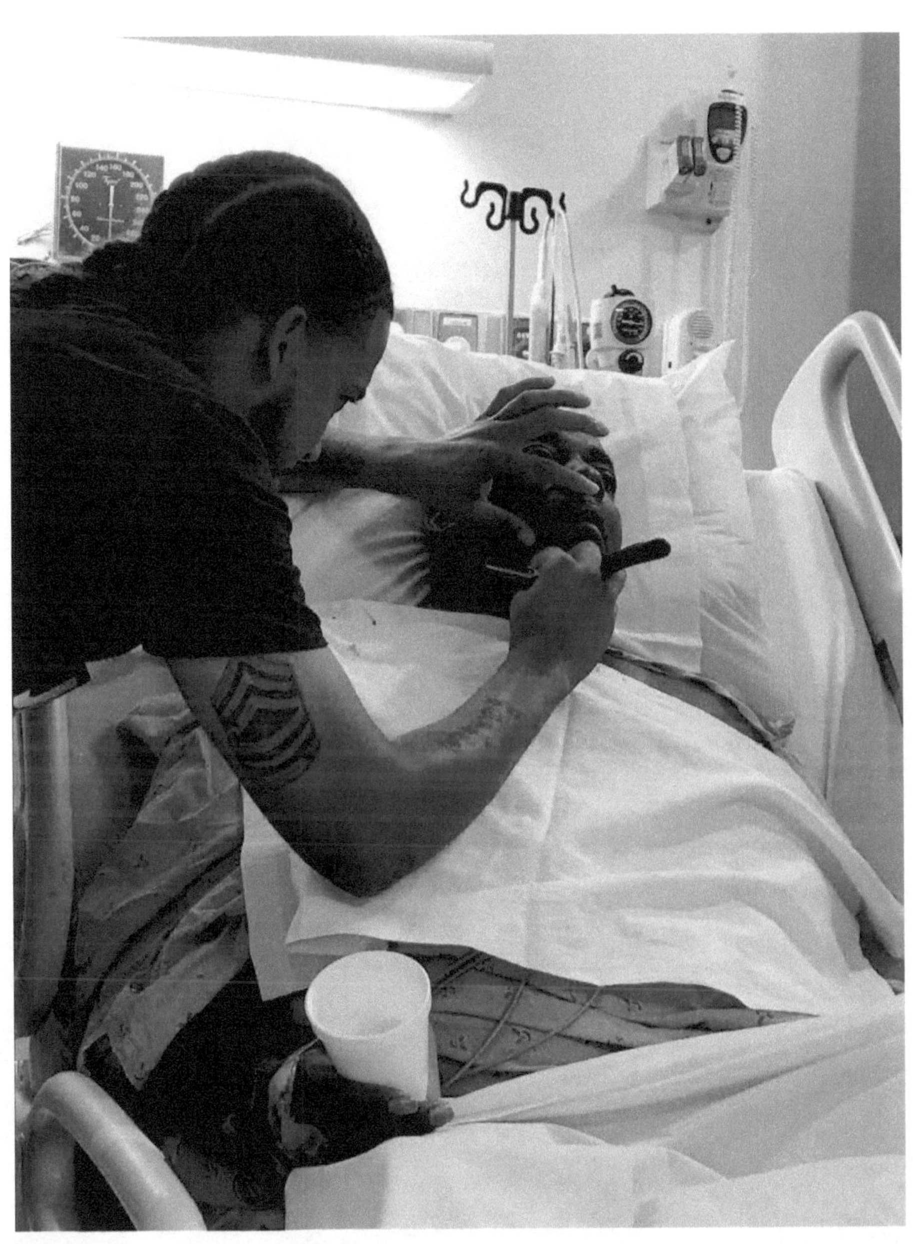

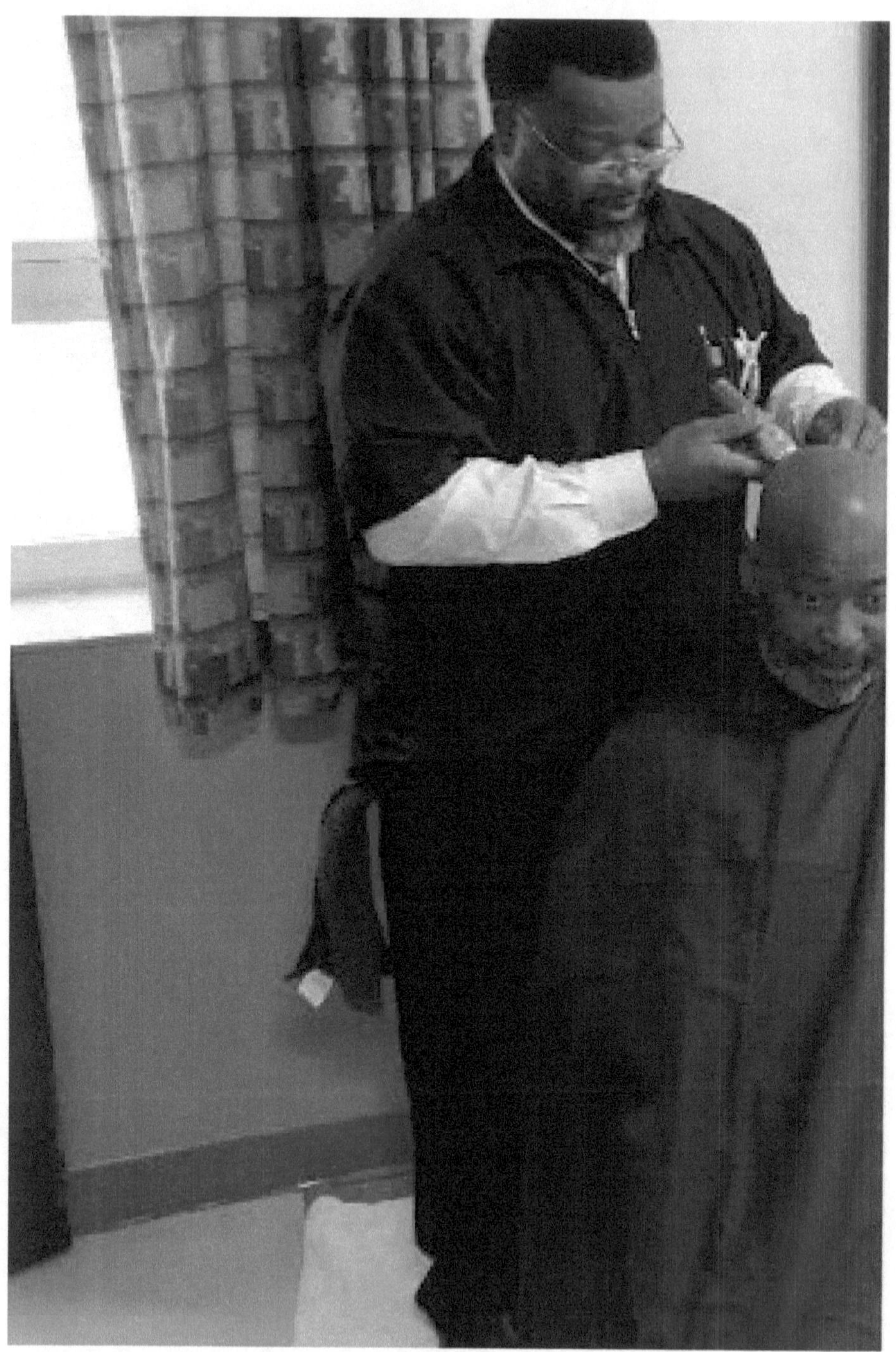

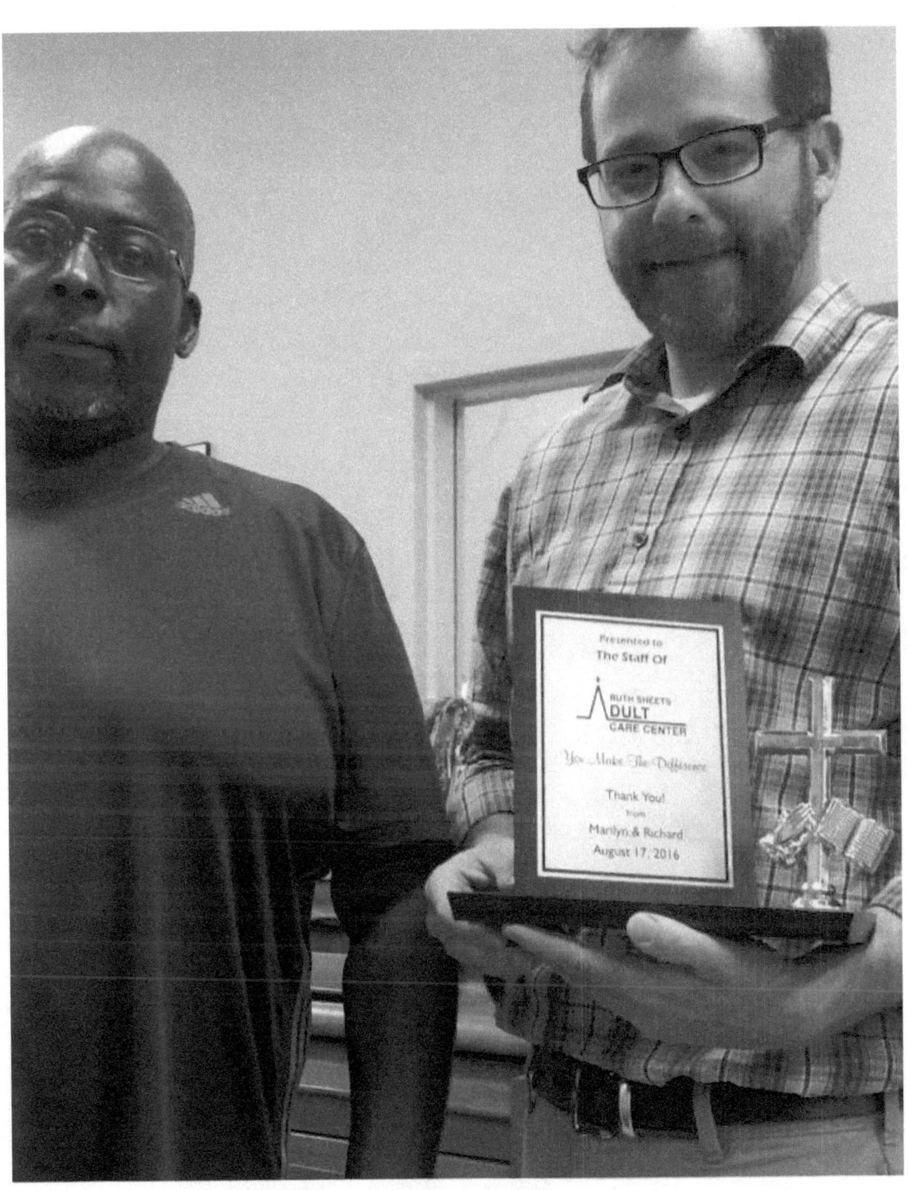

Presented to
The Staff Of
RUTH SHEETS
ADULT
CARE CENTER
You Make The Difference
Thank You!
from
Marilyn & Richard
August 17, 2016

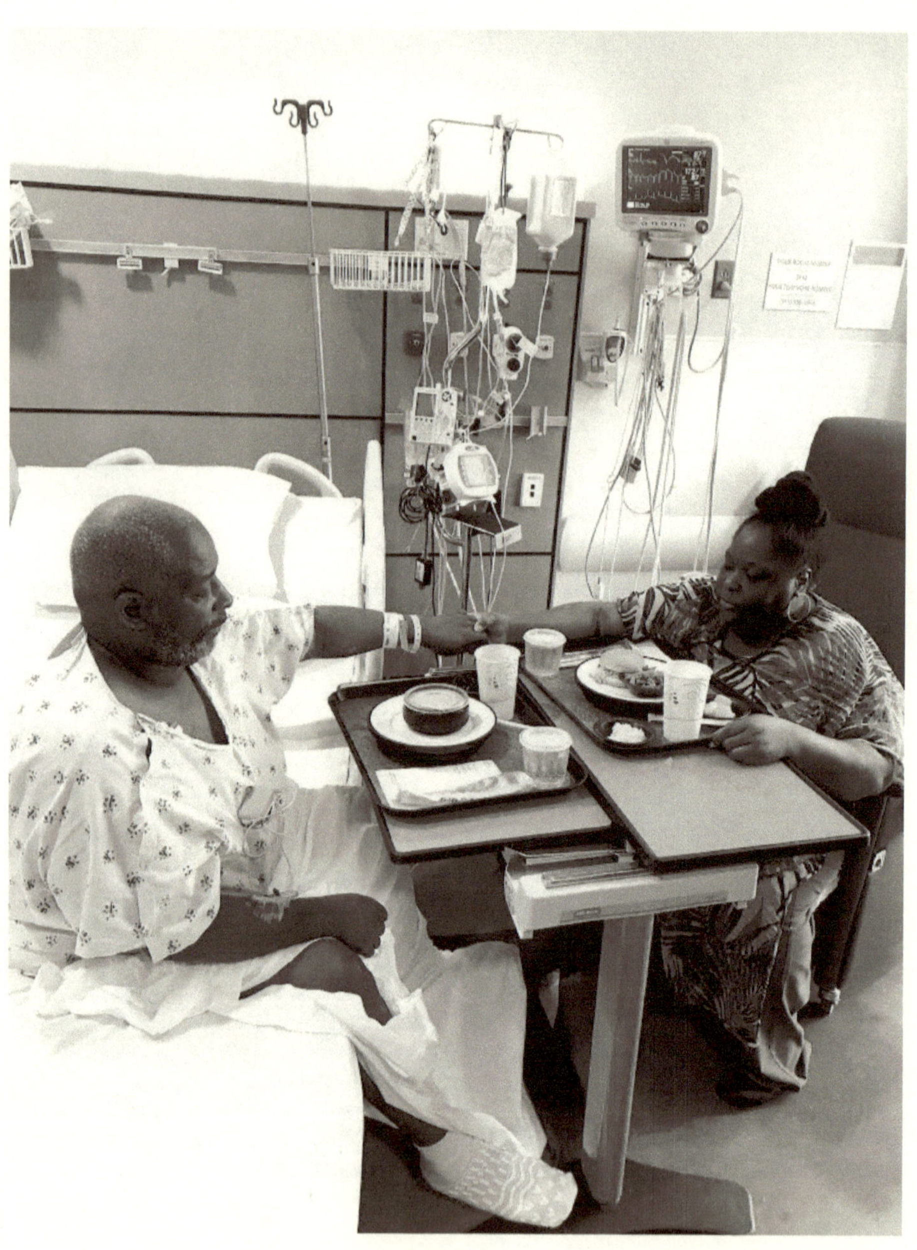

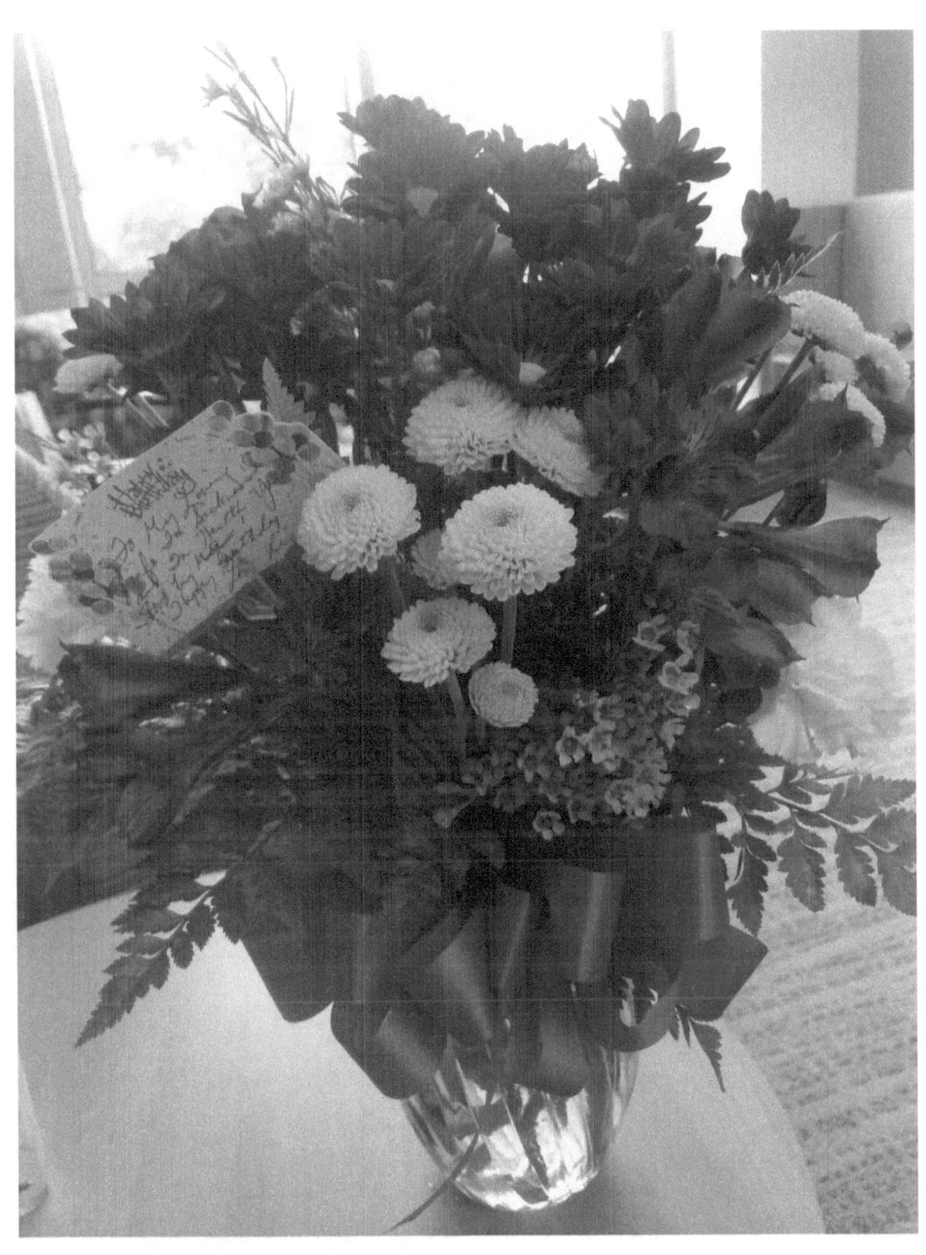

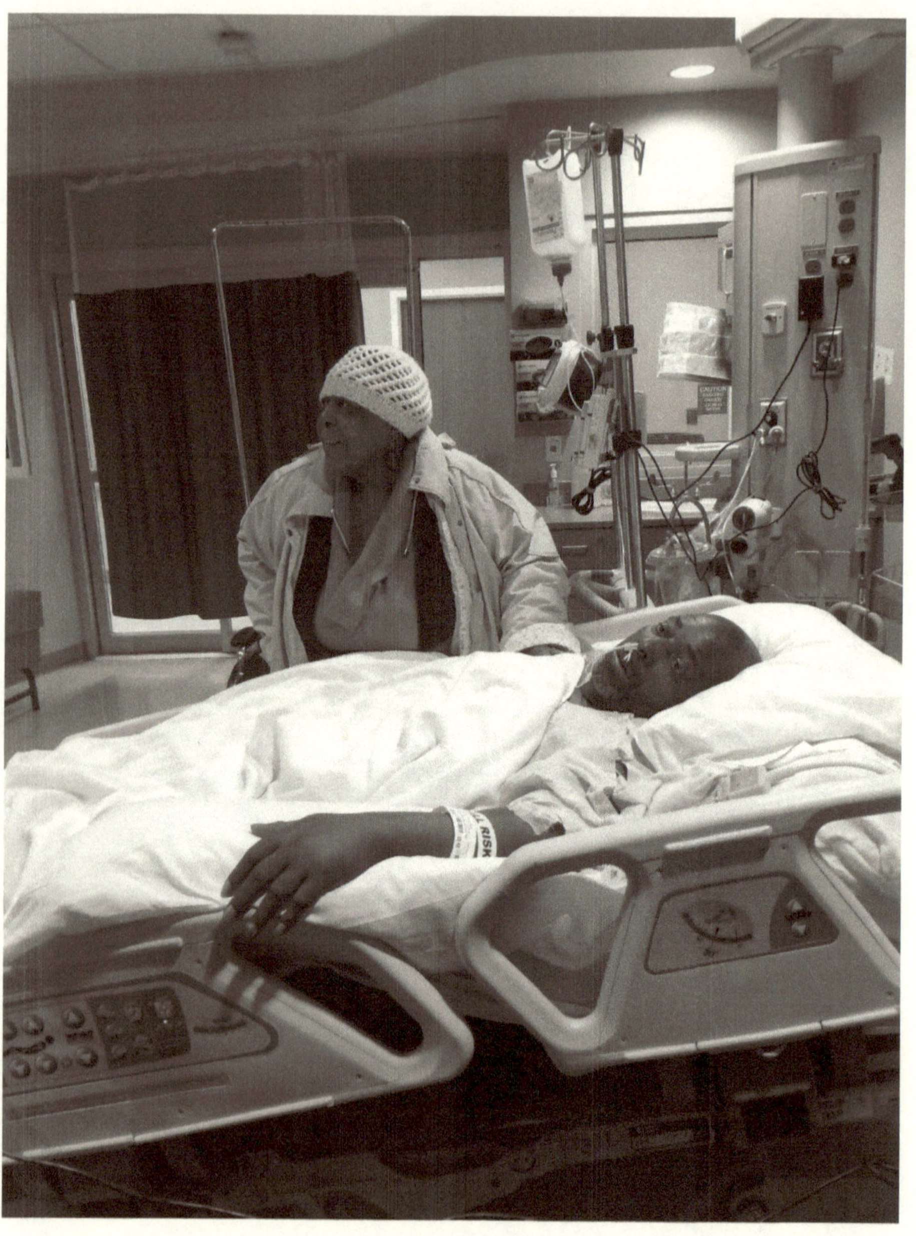

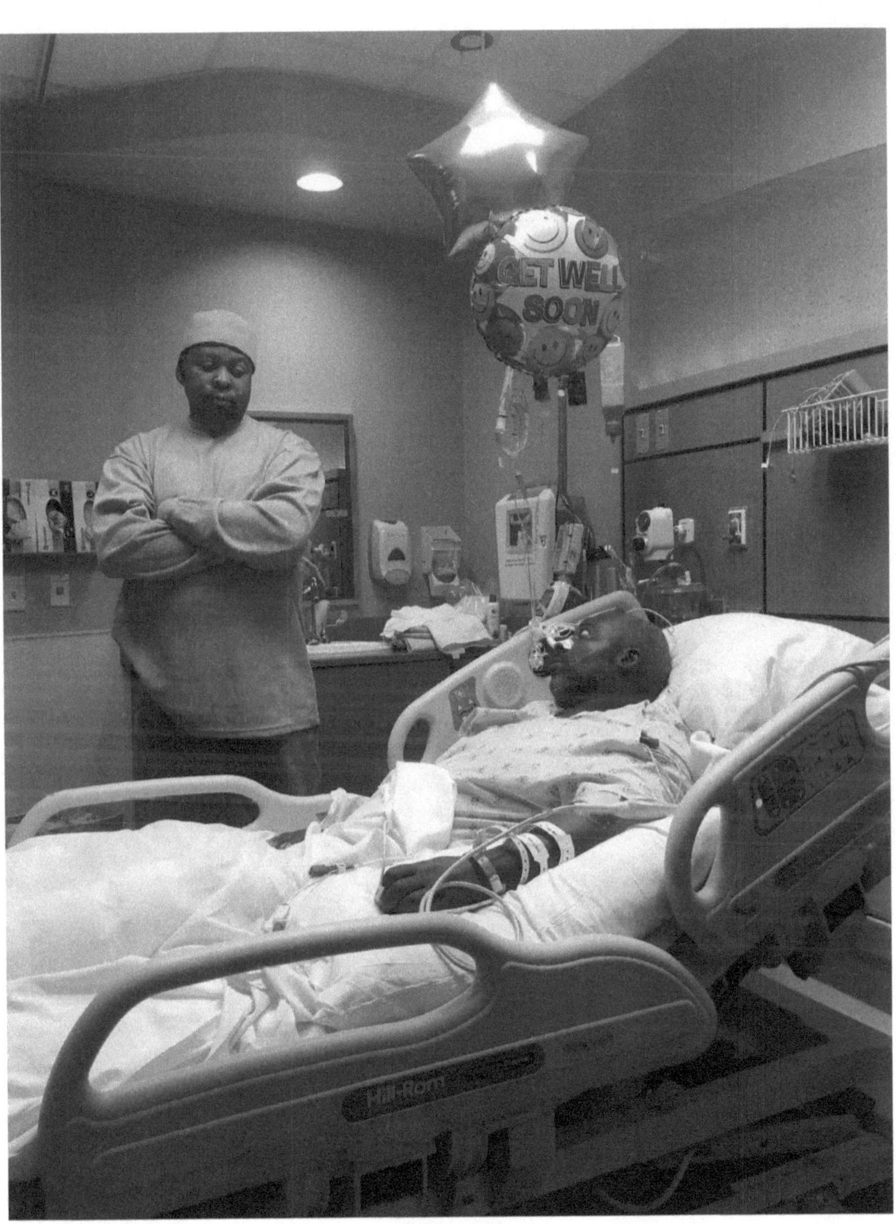

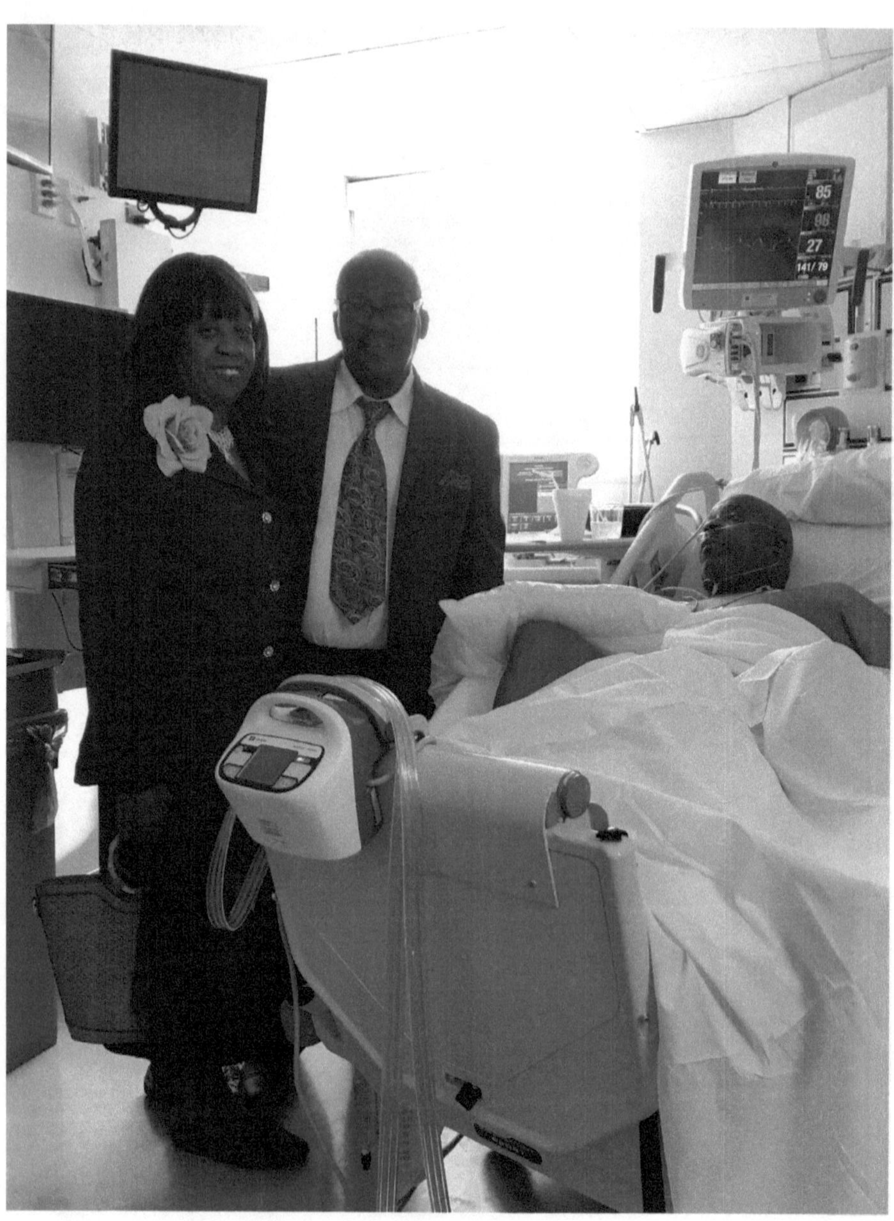

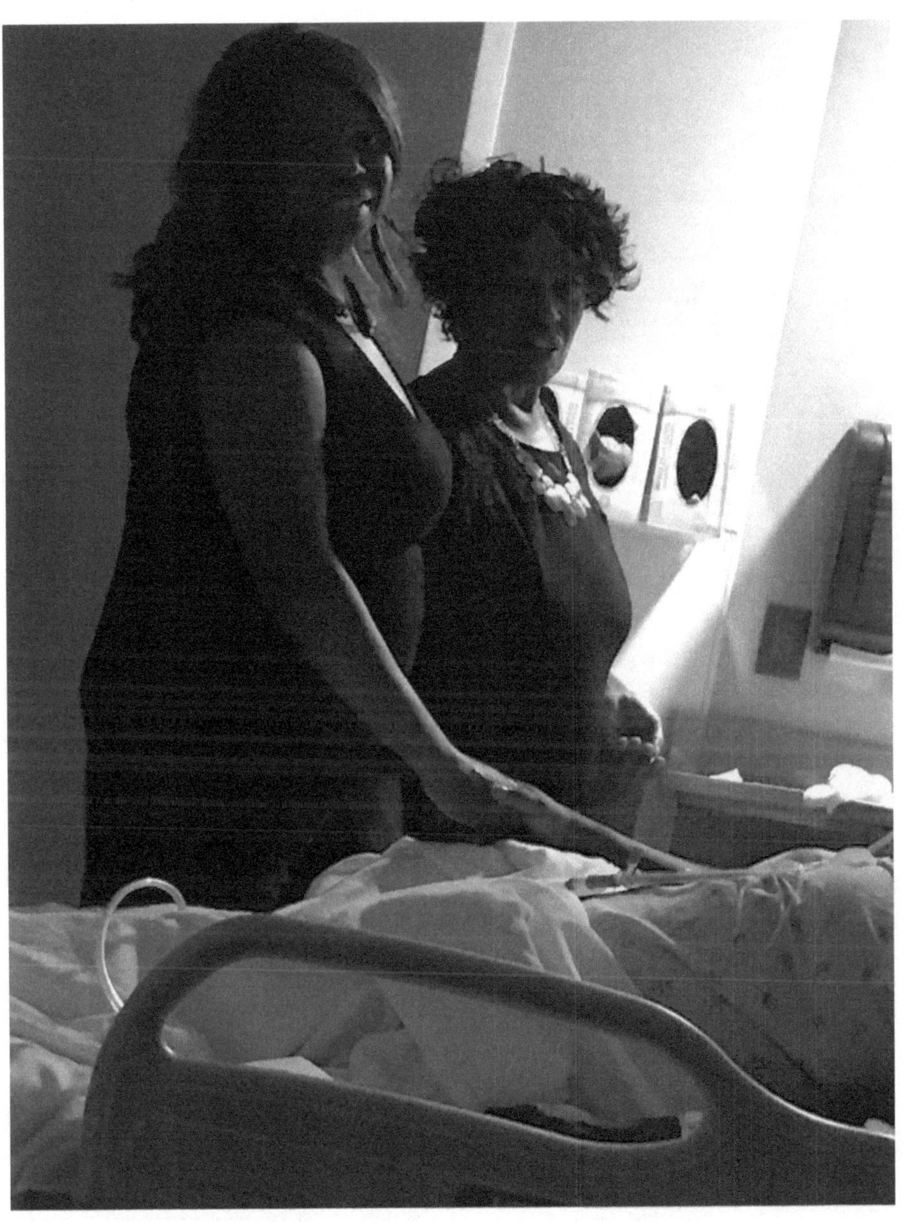

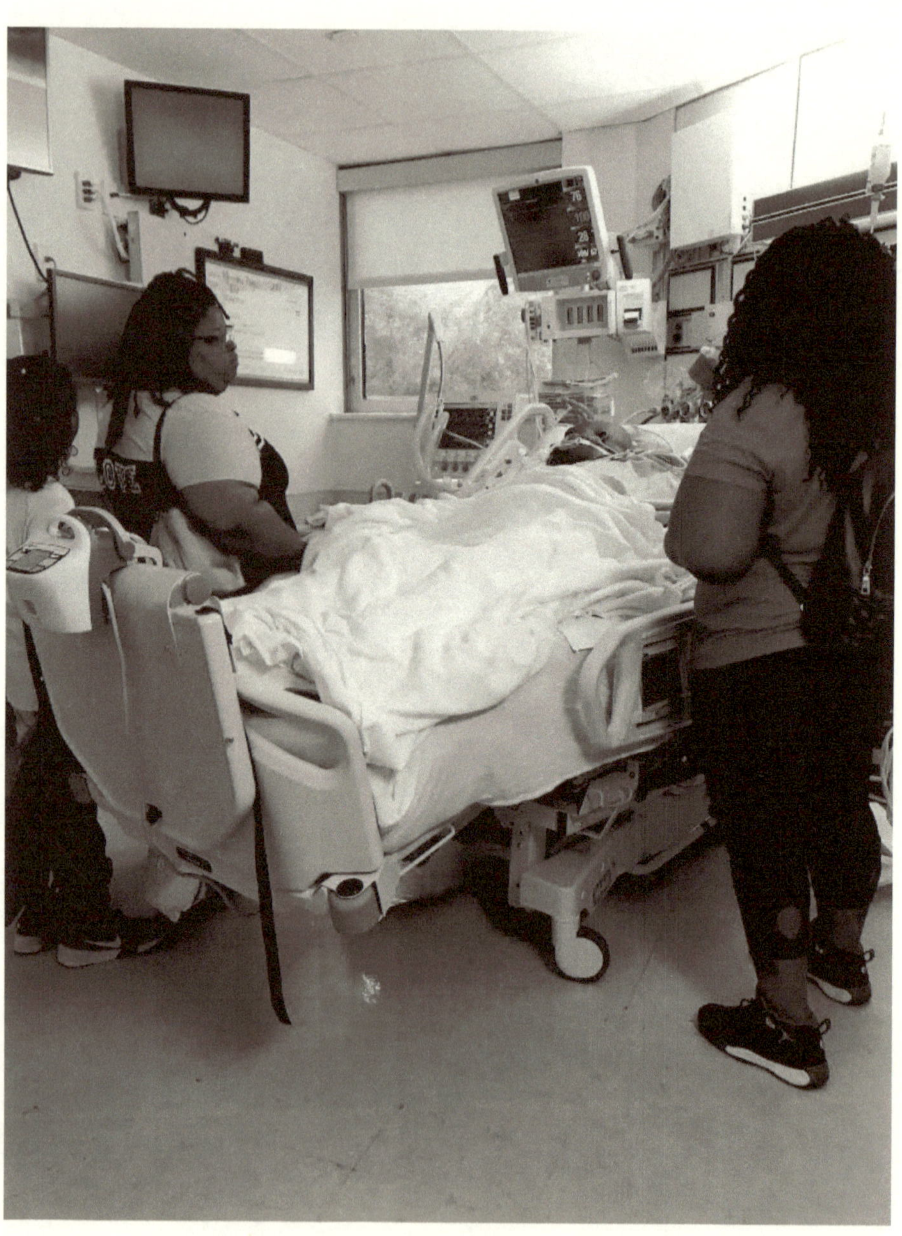

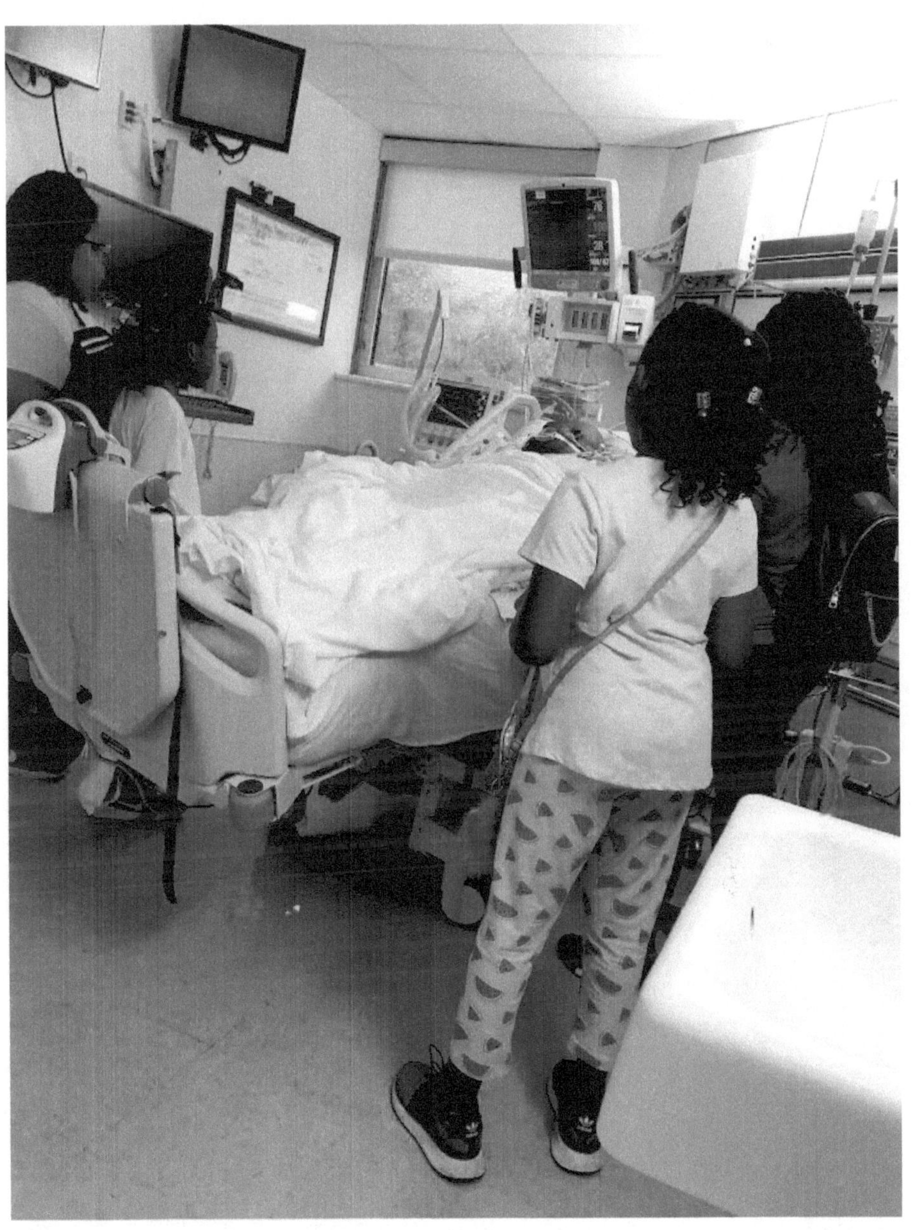

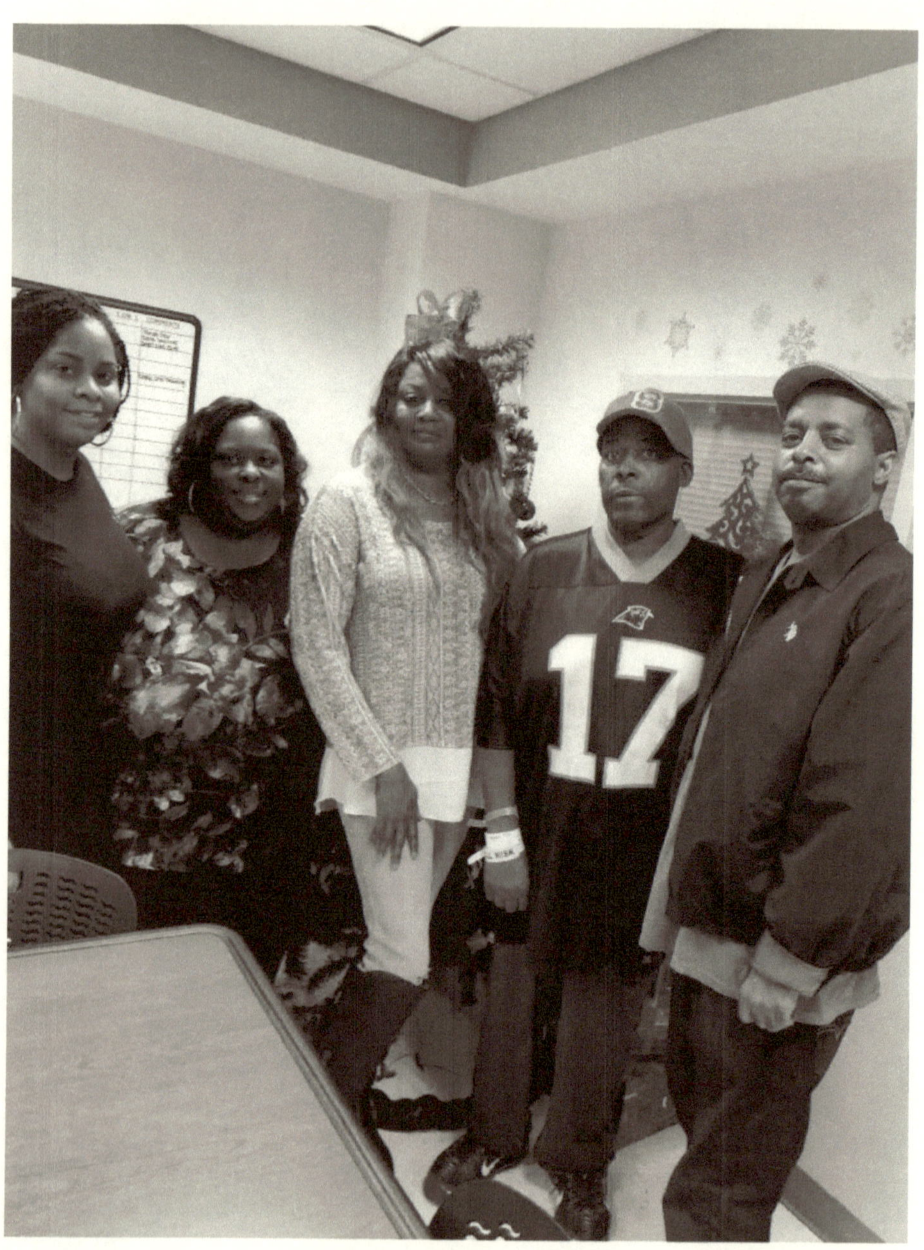

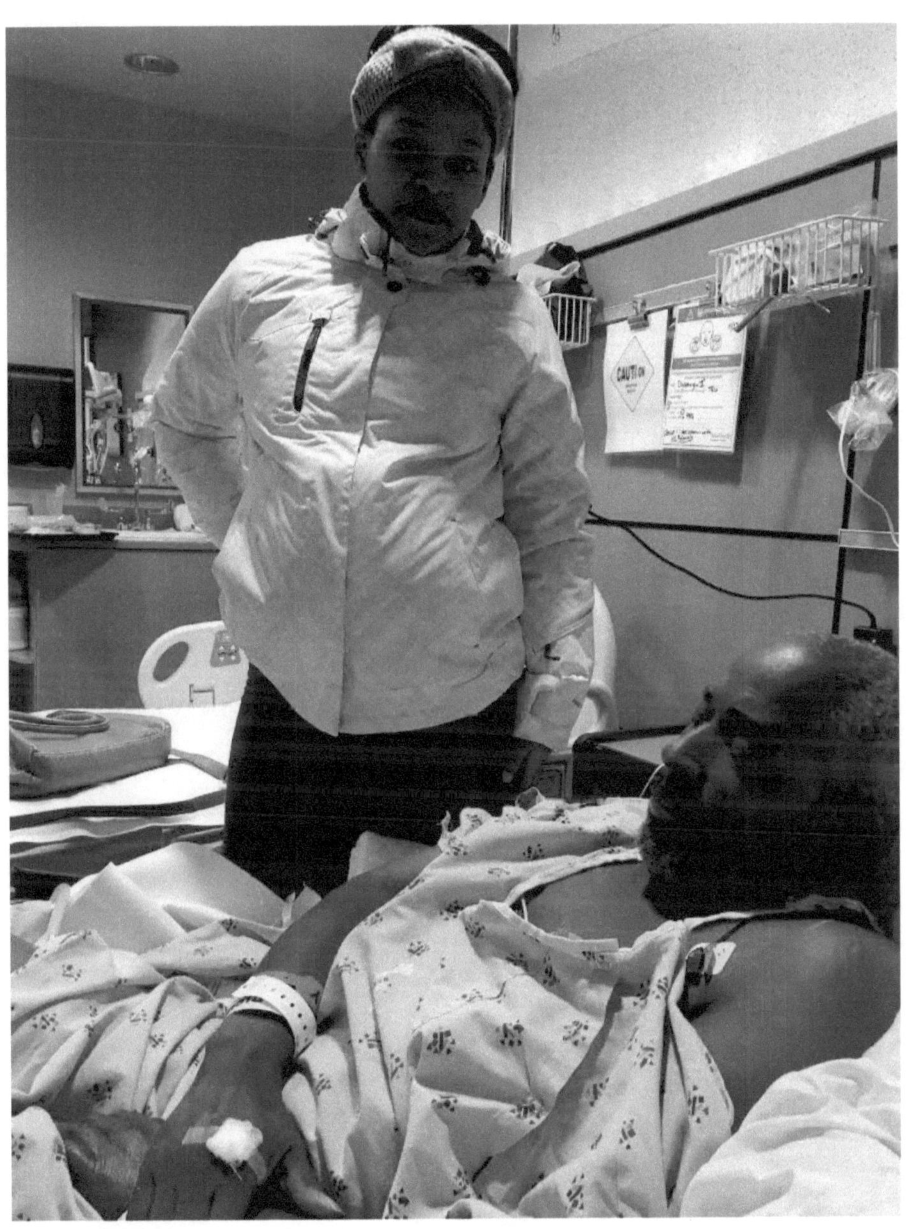

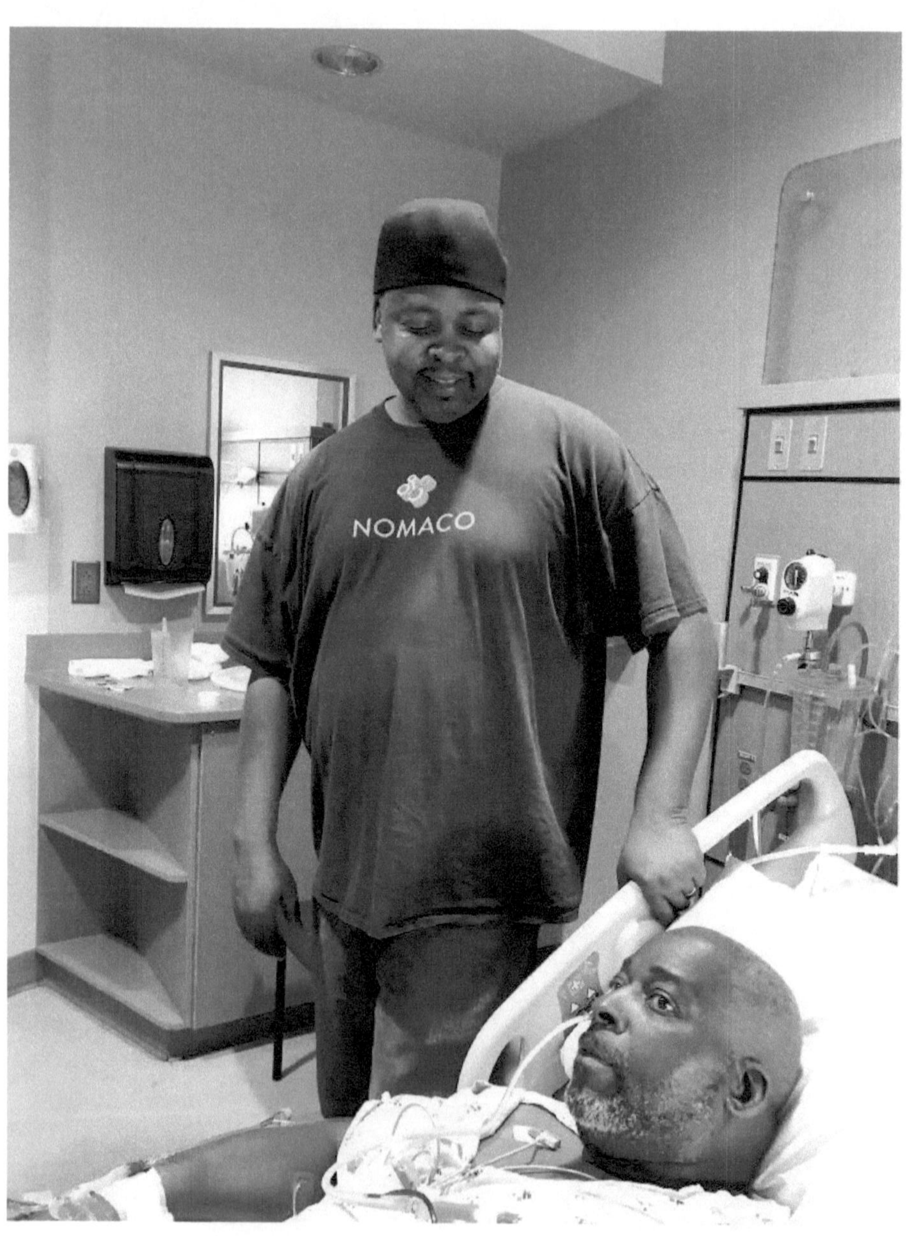

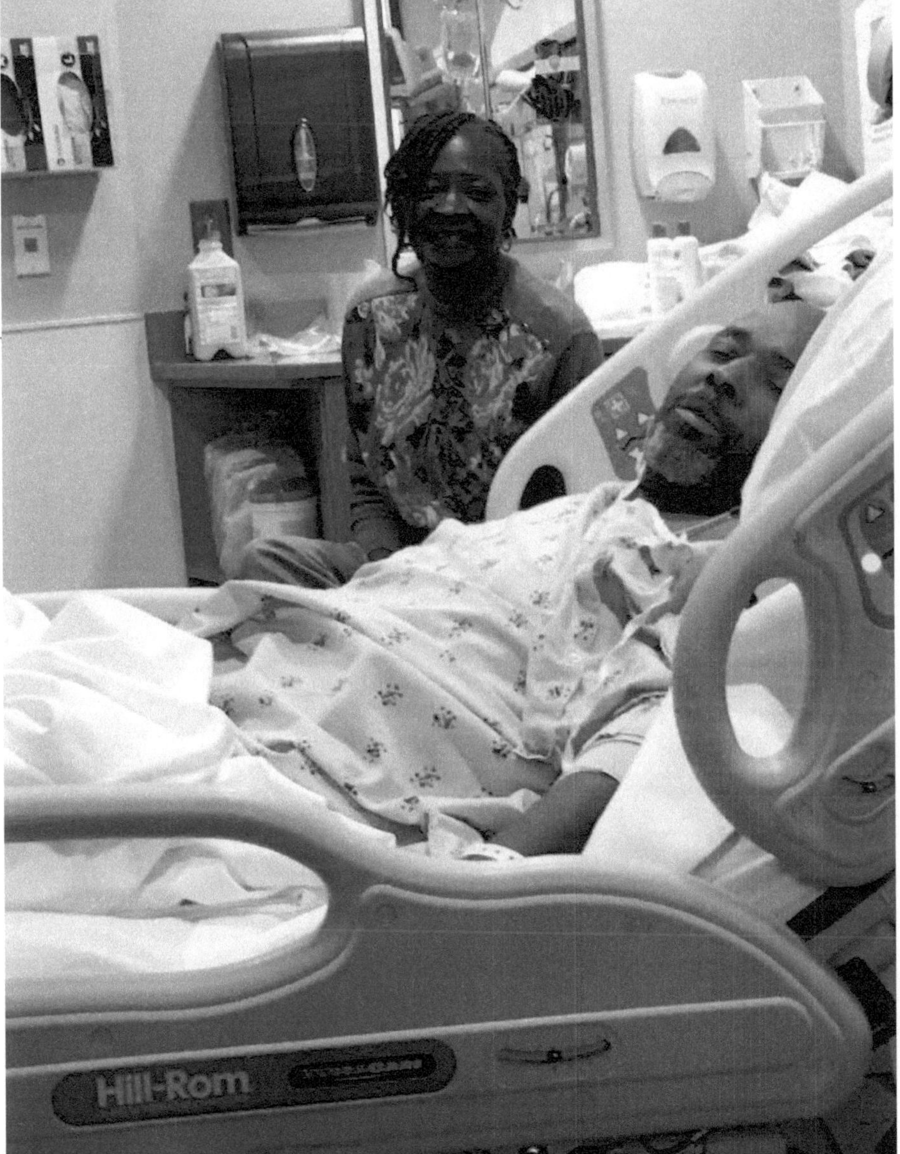

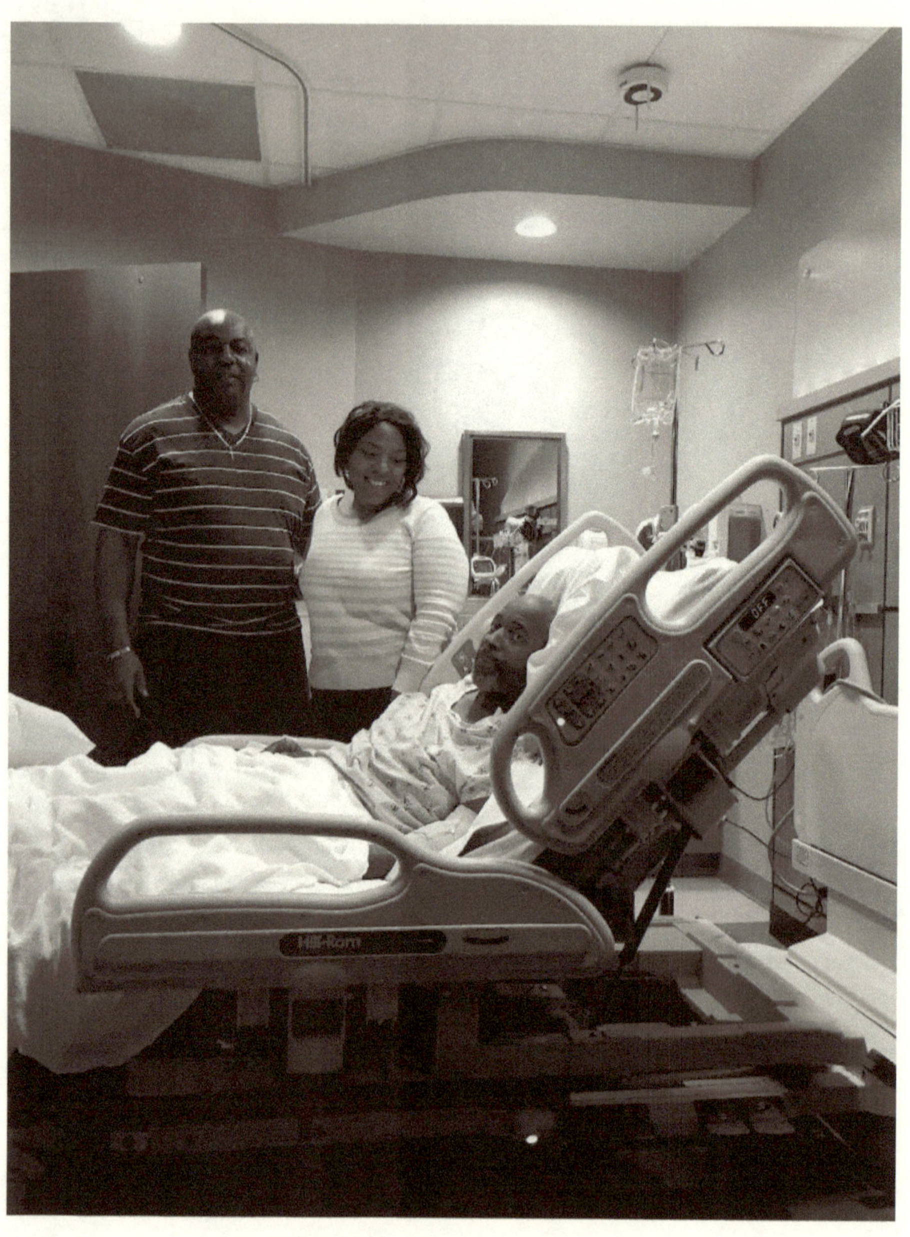

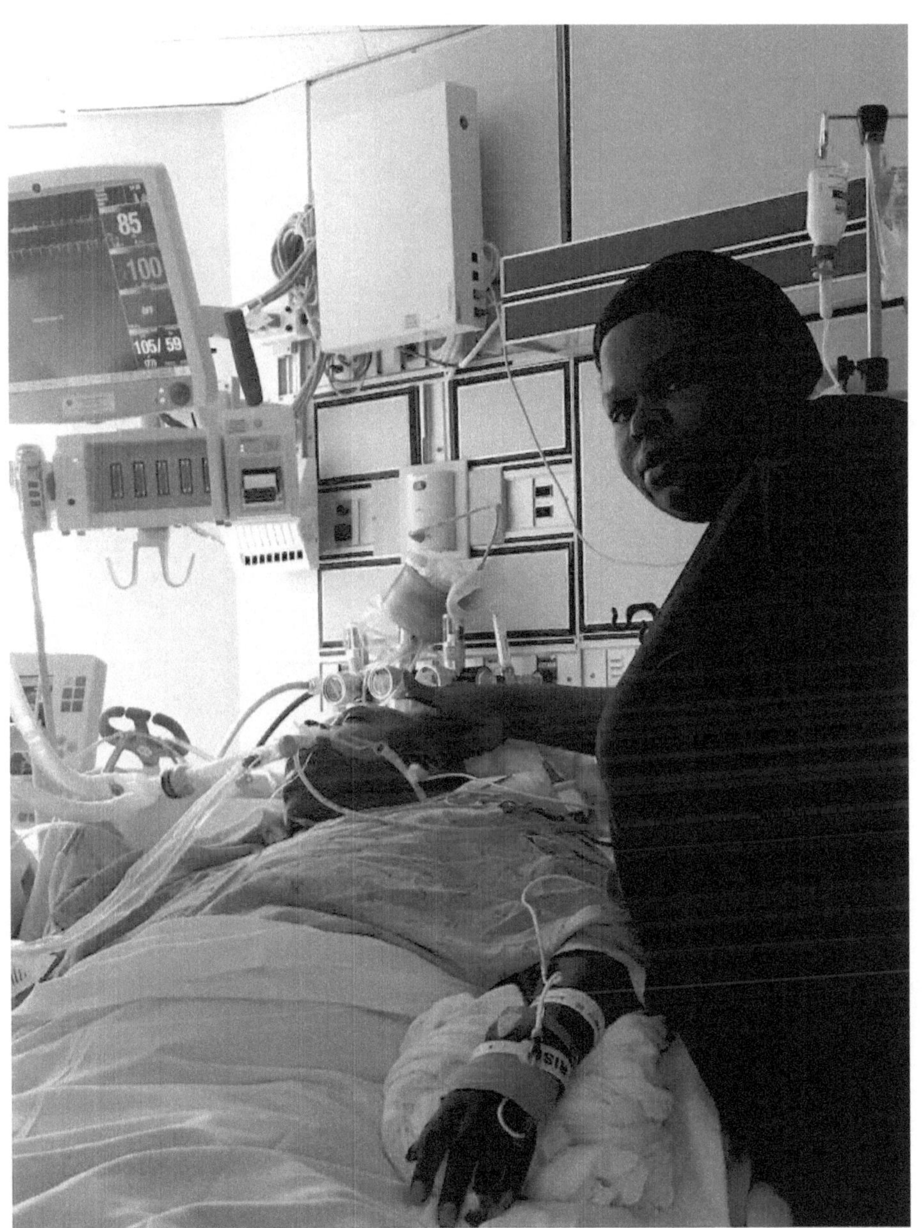

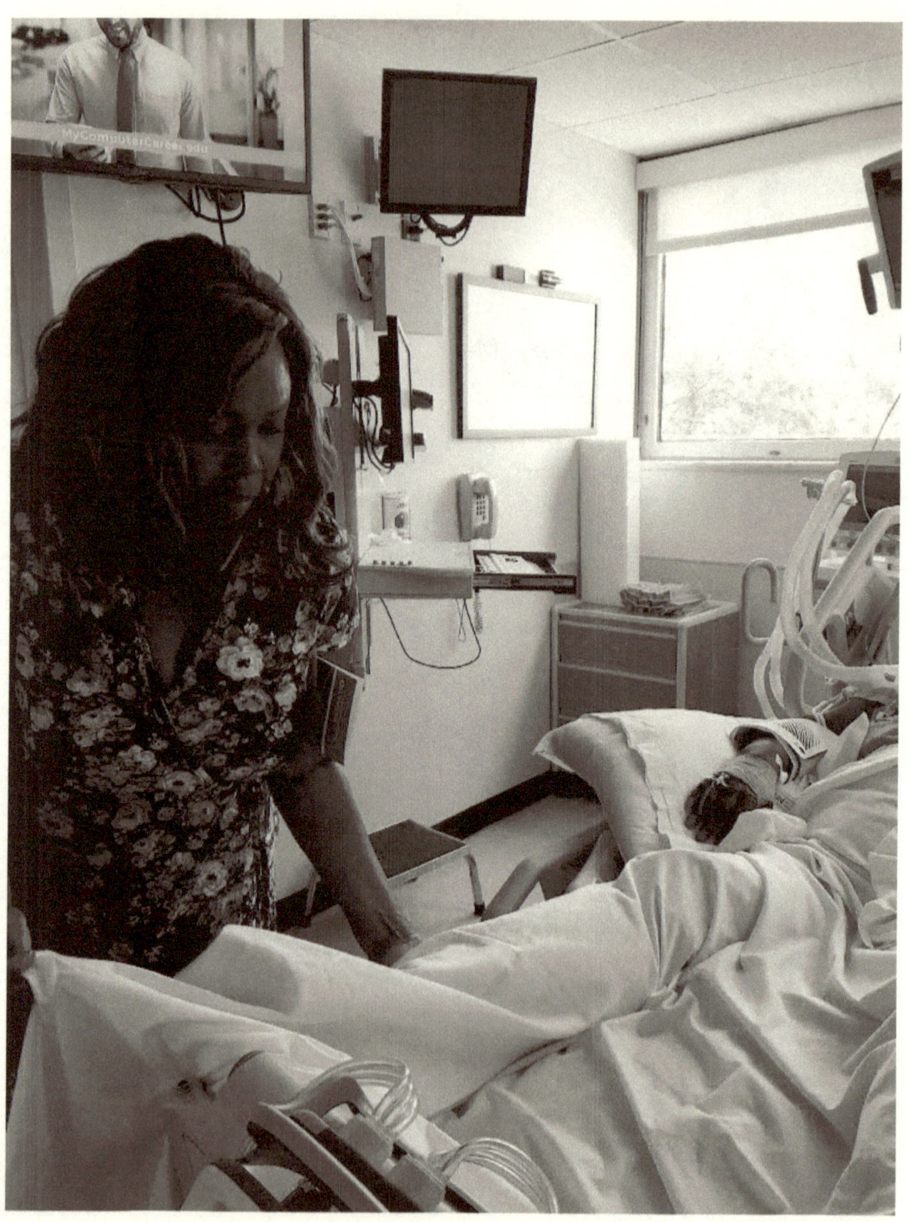

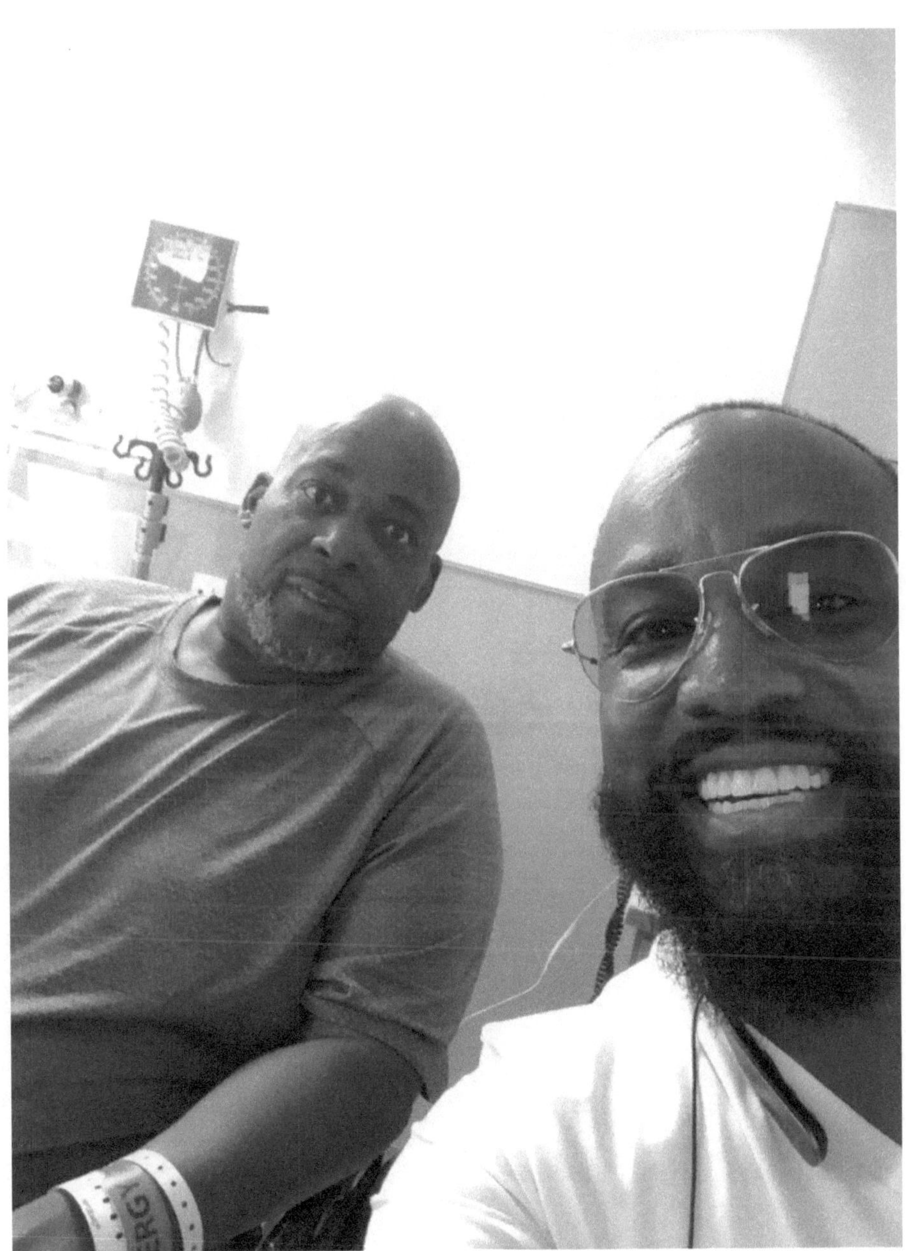

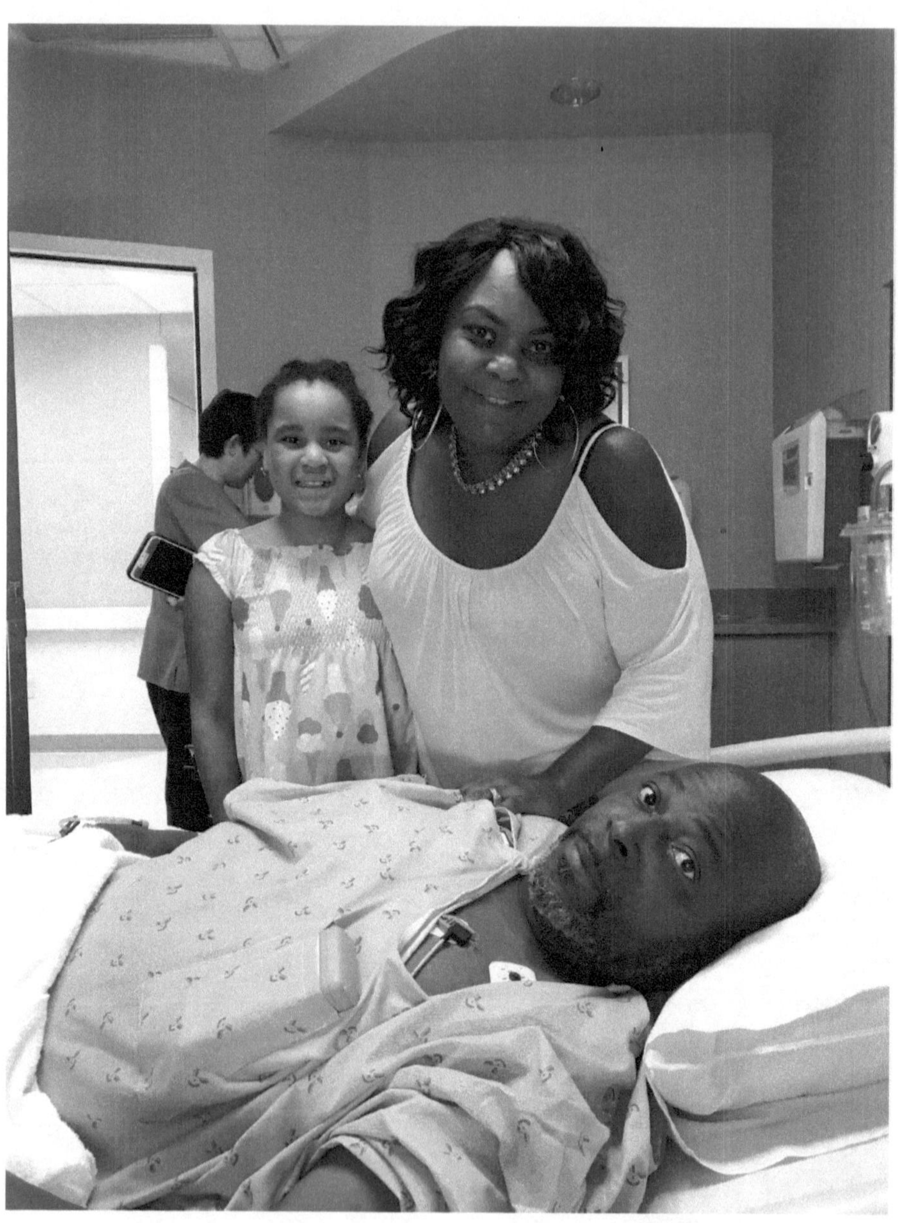

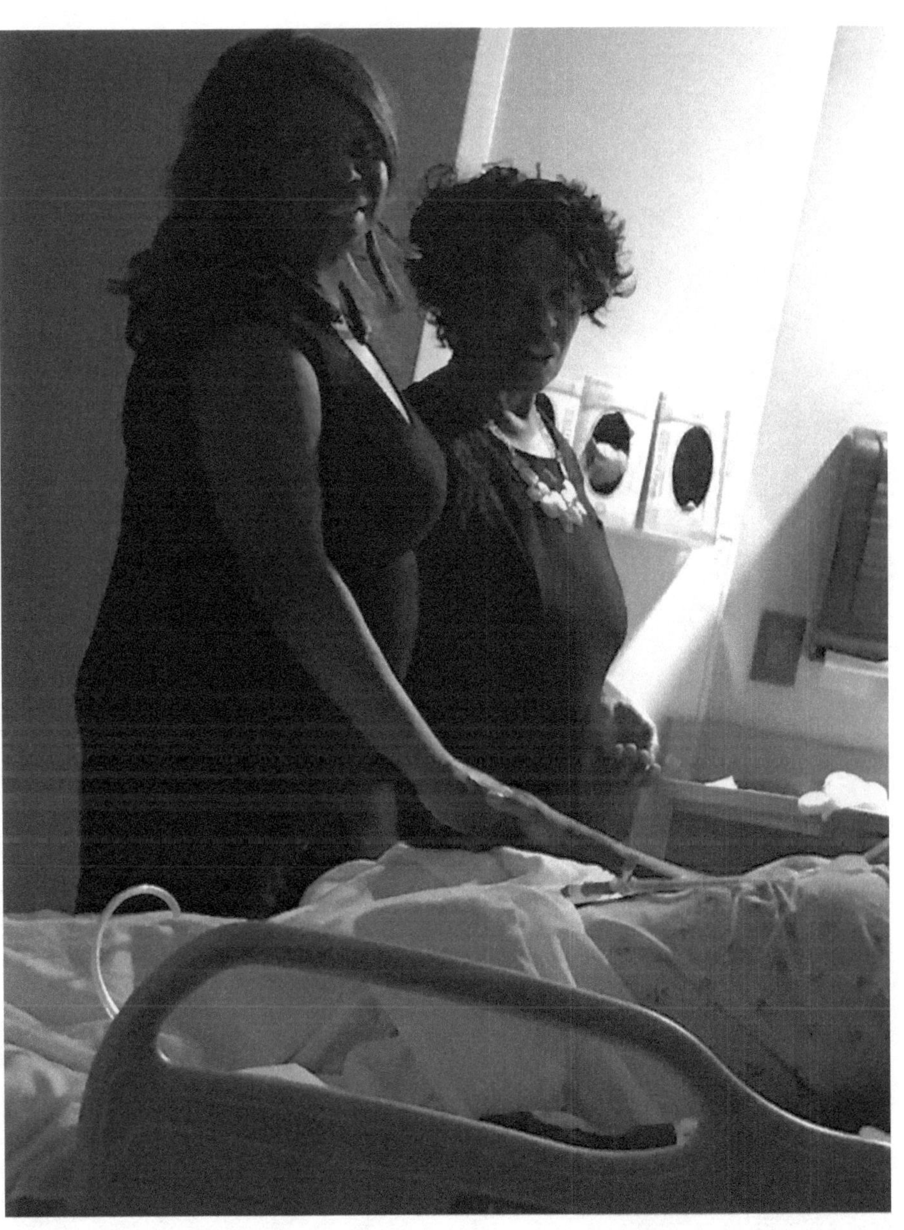

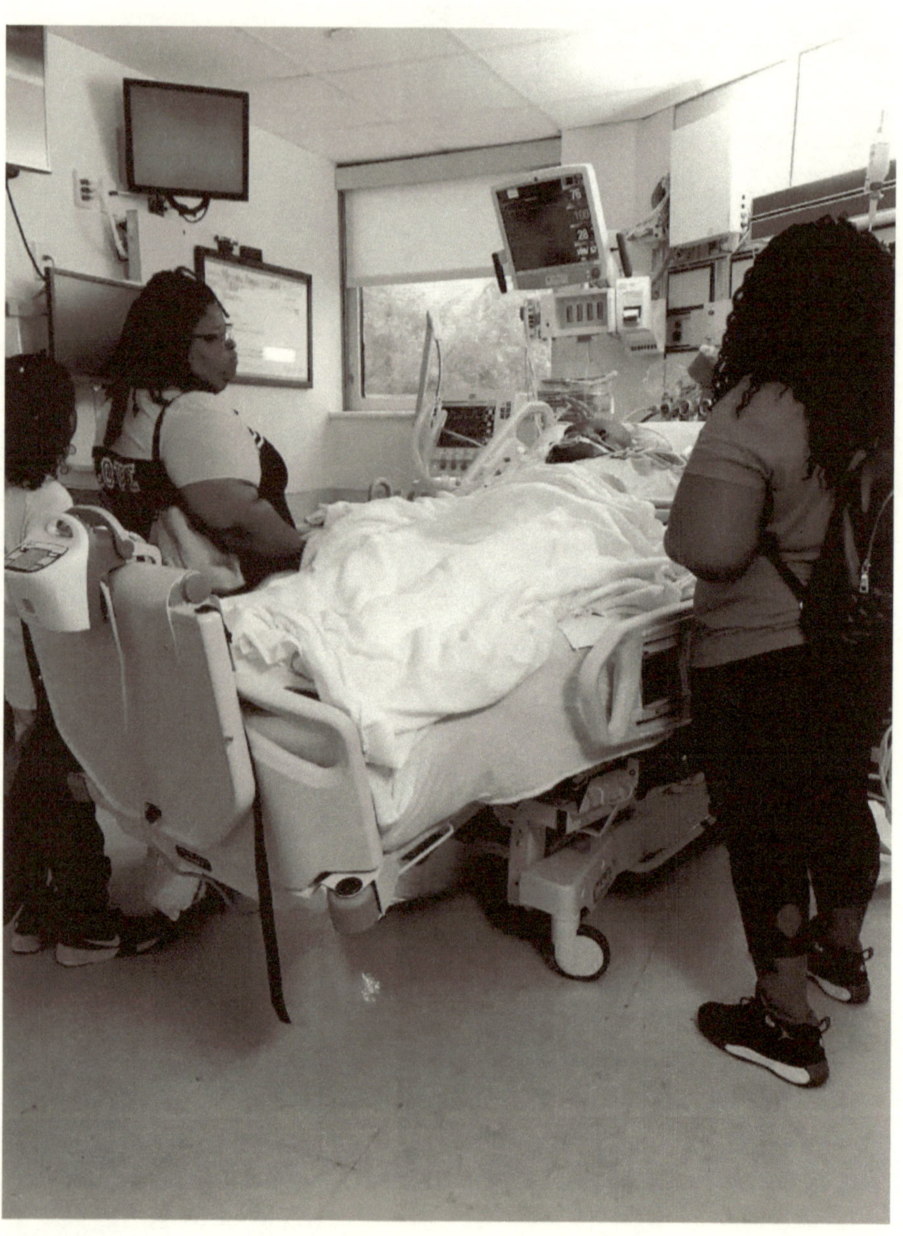

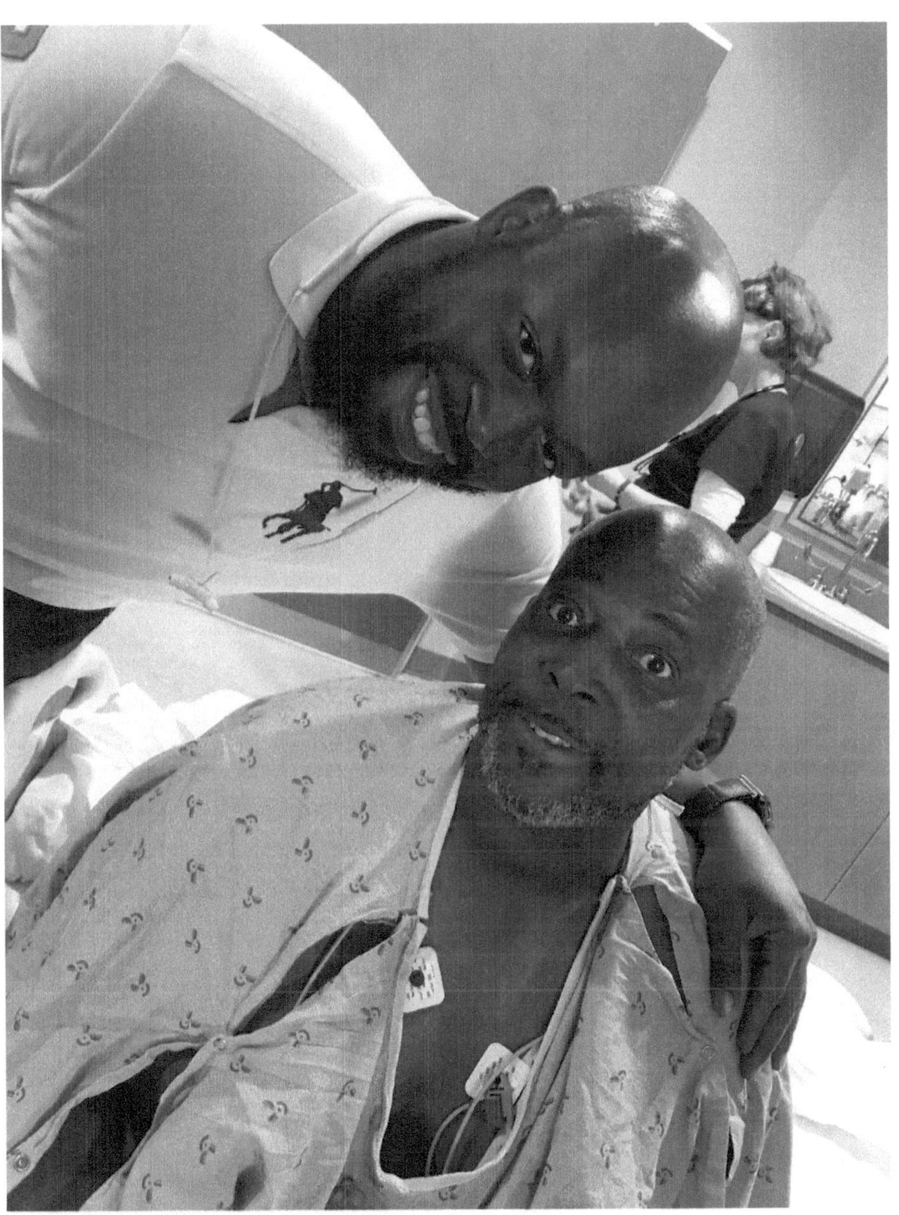

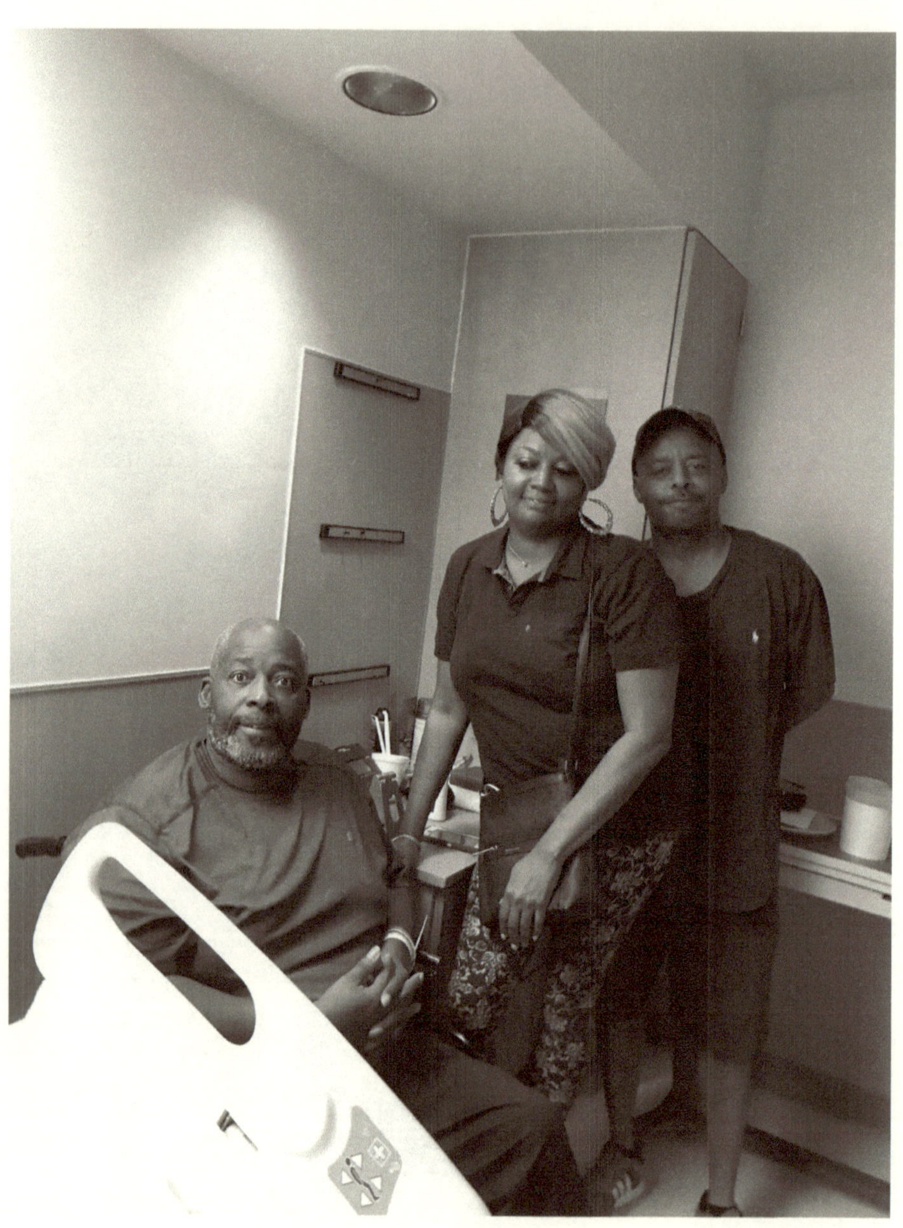

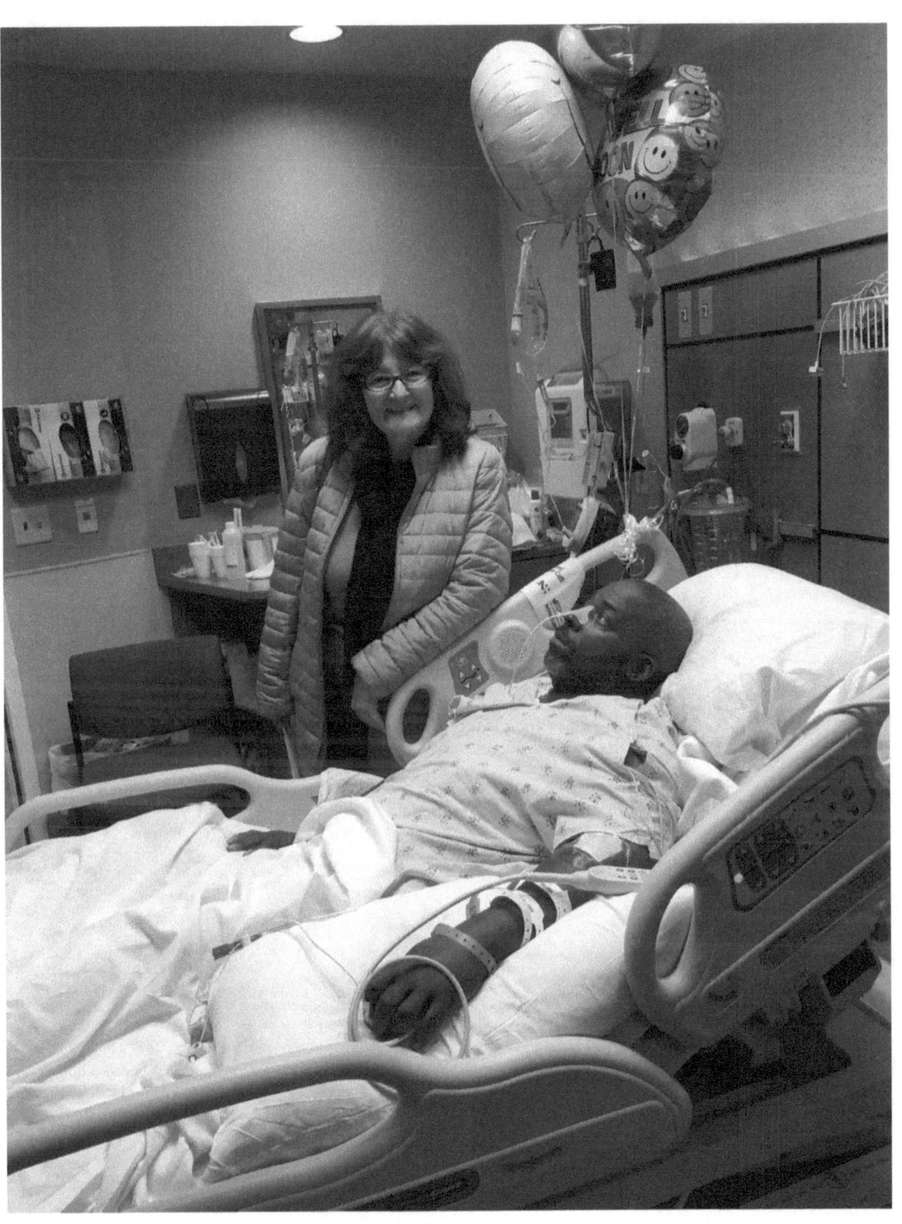

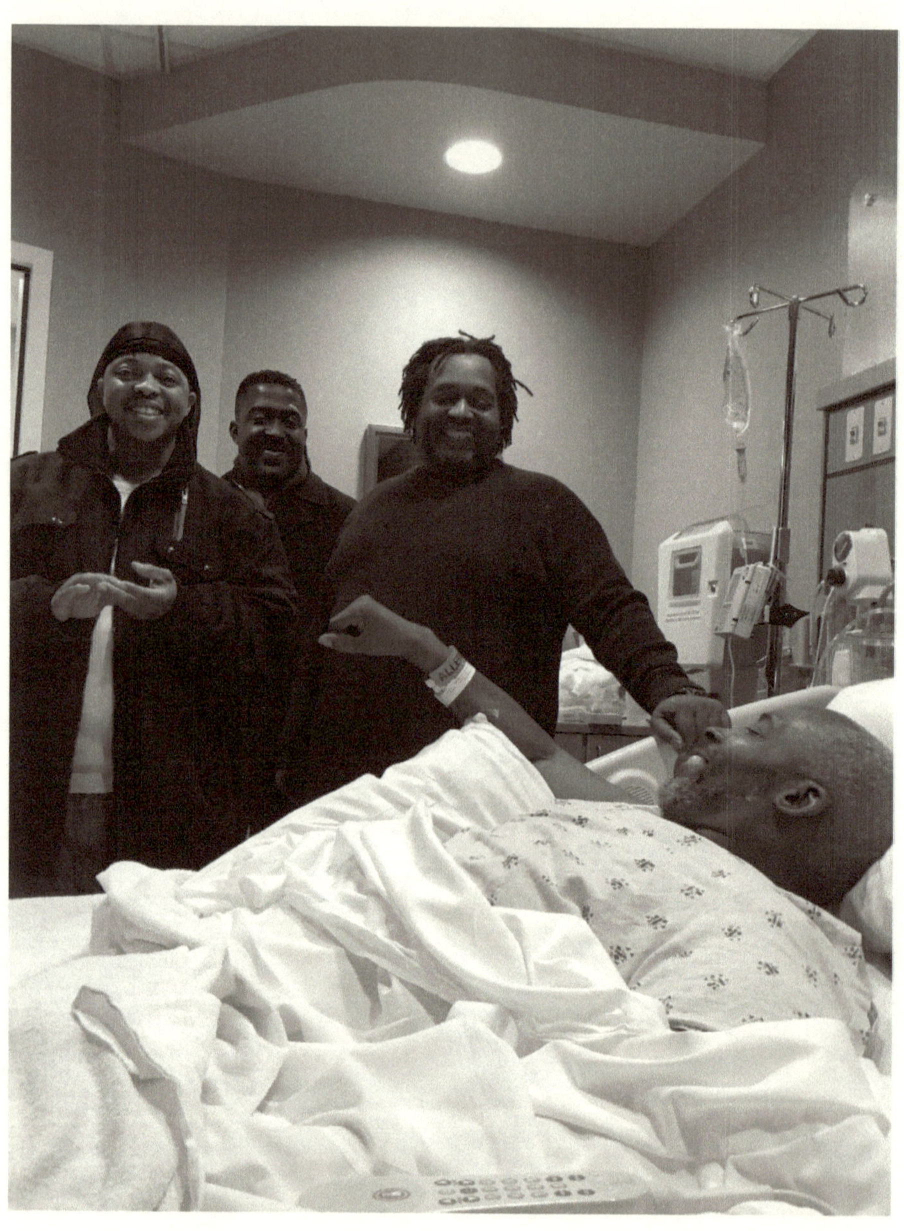

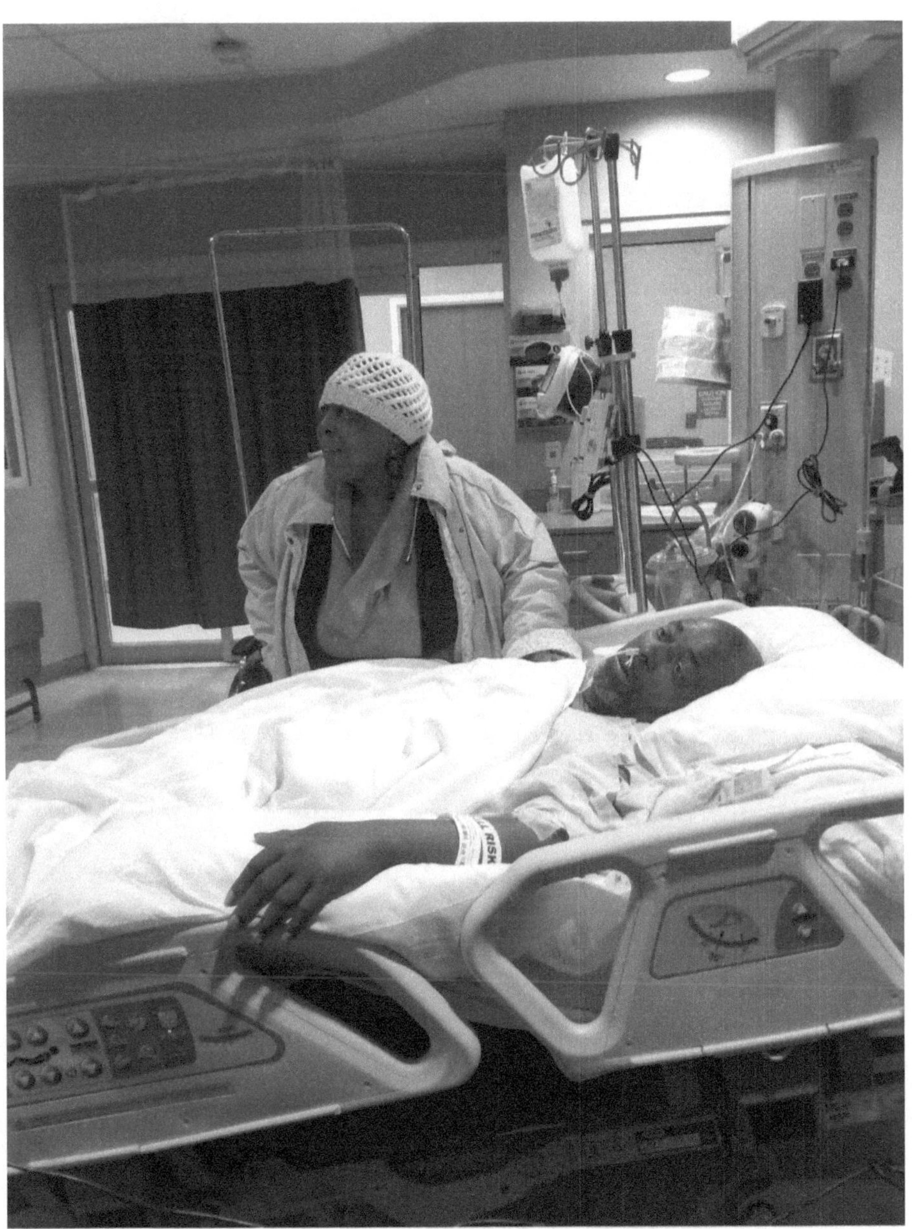

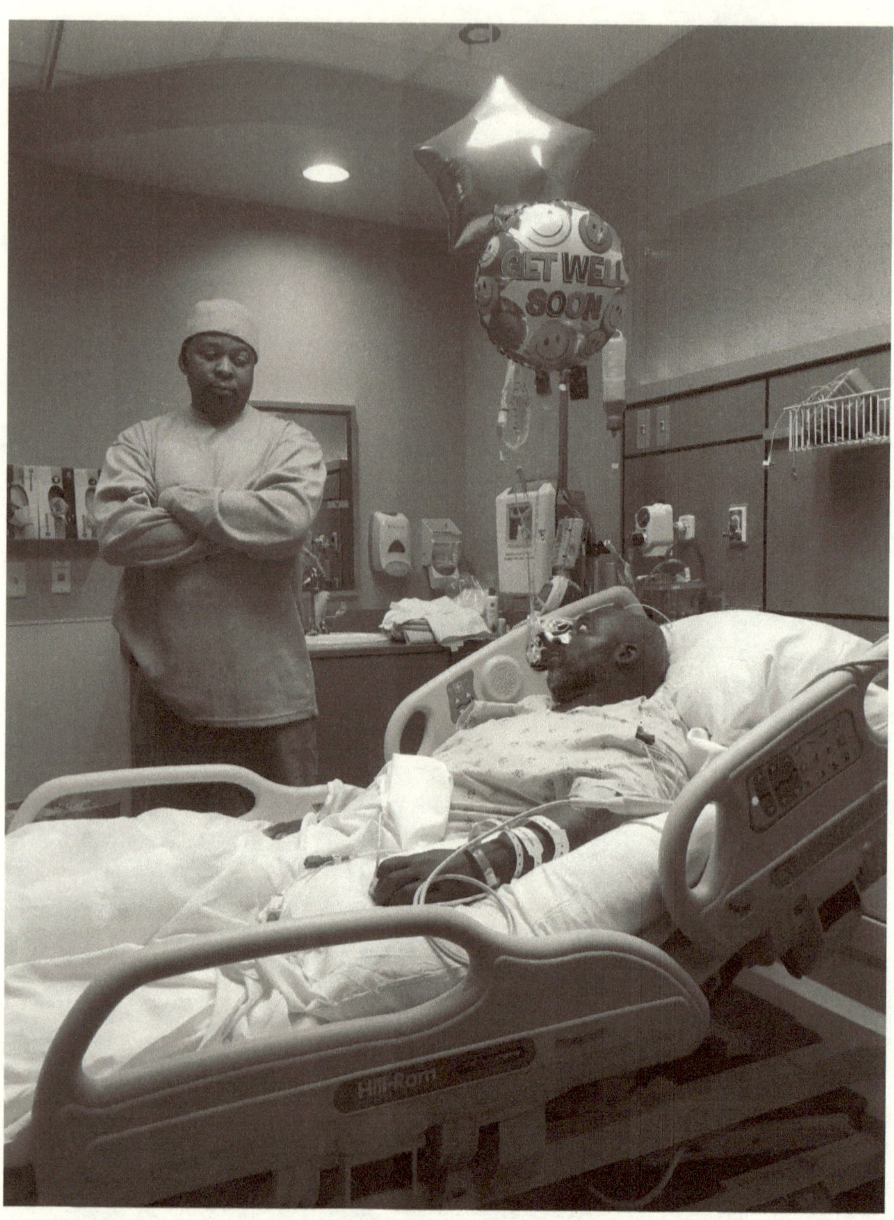

GET WELL
SOON
Hill-Rom

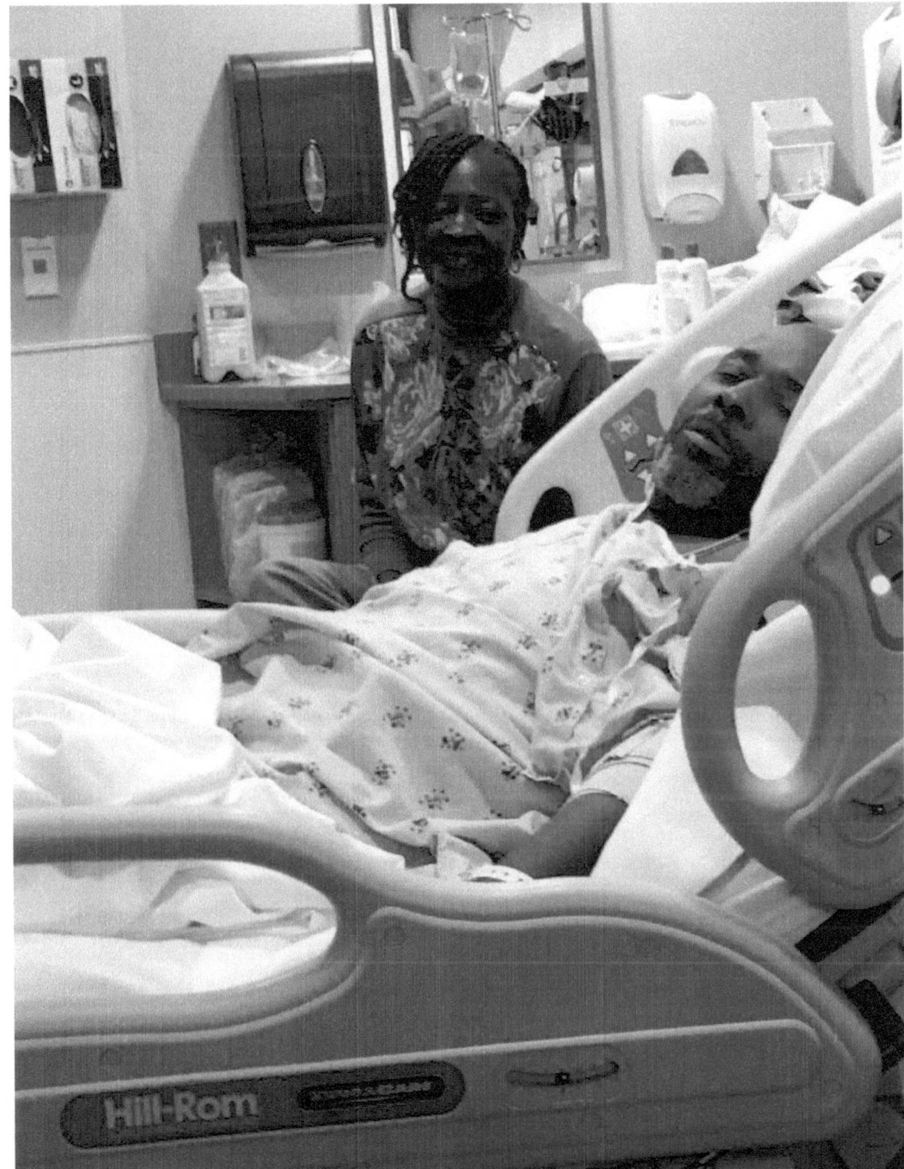

www.ingramcontent.com/pod-product-compliance
Lightning Source LLC
Chambersburg PA
CBHW051211250726
48655CB00006B/2349